A PATIENT'S GUIDE TO SURGERY

In Memory
Of
David Bird

Given By
Good Will
Hose Company
No. 2

A PATIENT'S GUIDE TO SURGERY

Edward L. Bradley III, M.D.
and the Editors of
Consumer Reports Books

CONSUMER REPORTS BOOKS
A Division of Consumers Union
Yonkers, New York

Published by Consumers Union of United States, Inc., Yonkers, New York 10703.

Library of Congress Cataloging-in-Publication Data
Bradley, Edward L.
A patient's guide to surgery / Edward L. Bradley III.
p. cm.
Includes index.
ISBN 0-89043-752-1
1. Surgery—Popular works. I. Title.
RD31.3.B73 1994
617—dc20
94-25995
CIP

Design by Abby Kagan

First printing, October 1994

This book is printed on recycled paper.

Manufactured in the United States of America

A Patient's Guide to Surgery is a Consumer Reports Book published by Consumers Union, the nonprofit organization that publishes *Consumer Reports*, the monthly magazine of test reports, product Ratings, and buying guidance. Established in 1936, Consumers Union is chartered under the Not-for-Profit Corporation Law of the State of New York.

The purposes of Consumers Union, as stated in its charter, are to provide consumers with information and counsel on consumer goods and services, to give information on all matters relating to the expenditure of the family income, and to initiate and to cooperate with individual and group efforts seeking to create and maintain decent living standards.

Consumers Union derives its income solely from the sale of *Consumer Reports* and other publications. In addition, expenses of occasional public service efforts may be met, in part, by nonrestrictive, noncommercial contributions, grants, and fees. Consumers Union accepts no advertising or product samples and is not beholden in any way to any commercial interest. Its Ratings and reports are solely for the use of the readers of its publications. Neither the Ratings, nor the reports, nor any Consumers Union publications, including this book, may be used in advertising or for any commercial purpose. Consumers Union will take all steps open to it to prevent such uses of its material, its name, or the name of *Consumer Reports*.

This book is dedicated to my patients, who have taught me life's true values, and to my wife, who has given me everything else

CONTENTS

A PATIENT'S GUIDE TO SURGERY

INTRODUCTION

This book is written for all surgical patients—past, present, and future. If you are like most people who learn they need surgery for the first time, you are unprepared for the experience and frightened about "going under the knife." Our intention is not only to help you prepare for the experience and assuage some of your fears but also to improve your chances for a successful outcome and enable you to recover more swiftly.

These goals can best be achieved by giving you the information you need to actively participate in all the important decisions required for a favorable surgical experience. If you don't take an active role in the surgical process, others will make the decisions that may be of critical importance to you. Although these decisions will be based on their ideas of what's best, even well-intentioned decisions by others may not be right for you.

Fortunately, the overwhelming majority of surgical operations performed in the United States each year are not emergencies; you can therefore take the opportunity to improve your chances for a successful surgical outcome by preparing yourself in advance.

Preparing yourself for surgery requires some of the same skills you use when making decisions about other aspects of daily life. You may have had to learn something about auto mechanics, gardening, home repair, or a host of other things: Does your transmission really need to be replaced? Can your lawn be saved? Should you invest in stocks now? If you're a conscientious consumer, you inform yourself on the topic and then hire advisers to help you make the right decisions. The decisions you need to make about surgery can be among the most important you'll ever make, and for these difficult choices you need absolutely reliable information.

This information may involve the quality of surgeons available in a prepaid health plan, so you can make an intelligent choice among competing plans. It's not enough just to compare costs—you need to evaluate the qualifications of the physicians themselves. Of course, financial considerations are a strong secondary concern.

It is an unfortunate truth that inadequate and inappropriate surgery is performed every day in this country. In just one year, surgeons have operated on the wrong eye, the wrong leg, the wrong side of the brain, and even the wrong patient. Although it's true such inexcusable incidents are rare, the fact remains that they do happen and they could happen to you. Without question, there are bad surgeons at work. Fortunately, you or someone close to you may be able to avoid them. This can be accomplished by working closely with your family doctor (or even by yourself, if you so choose) to materially affect many of the decisions regarding a proposed operation.

In these pages you'll learn how to evaluate alternatives to surgery, why preoperative testing is necessary, how to choose a surgeon and the appropriate form of anesthesia, what the day of surgery is like, what you can and cannot expect from surgery, how quality control in surgery is maintained, and many other considerations of critical importance.

With this book you can also remove the shroud of mystery that envelops the surgical experience and the profession of surgery. Best of all, armed with the information contained in this book, you may be able to save yourself, or those you love, from the considerable suffering and expense of a bad surgical experience.

WHY YOU NEED THIS BOOK

In 1992, more than 25 million Americans underwent surgery. Statistically speaking, your chances of having an operation this year are roughly 1 in 10. Fortunately, 4 out of every 5 operations performed in the United States are not emergency procedures. This means that there's usually plenty of time before an operation must be scheduled in which to consider your options and improve your chances for successful surgery by learning something about surgery and surgeons.

There are a few things people can do to improve their overall physical health. We all know the basic ones: eat a low-cholesterol diet, drink alcohol in moderation, cut out all tobacco, and exercise regularly. Now you can add another to this list: Protect yourself from bad surgery.

Do you really need to protect yourself? In a 1990 study of more than 30,000 patients randomly chosen from 51 New York State hospitals, researchers found that 4 out of every 100 patients were actually harmed while under care in the hospital. Of those who were harmed, 14 percent died as a result of negligence and more than half of those harmed were victims of surgical errors.

SURGERY IS AN ART, NOT A SCIENCE

Be assured that the overwhelming majority of surgeons are competent and dedicated. But what if you're unlucky enough to find a bad one?

Despite constant effort, a great deal of surgery remains an art rather than a science. The word *science* is derived from the Latin word meaning "to know." However, in the everyday practice of surgery, many decisions must be made without "knowing" absolutely that the decision is the correct one. This is because so much remains unknown about the human body and how it reacts to illness and injury. Surgeons fill in the gaps in scientific knowledge with educated guesses based on their experience. Those guesses are called "surgical judgment." It is in the application of surgical judgment that a large part of surgery becomes an art.

Of course, the better surgeons have more control over the science aspect, which helps them to reach correct judgments. But only when both scientific knowledge and surgical judgment are properly applied to the care of patients are the best results achieved.

THE LOGIC OF SURGICAL ERRORS

Most of the bad surgery performed in this country is far less dramatic than glaringly obvious mistakes, such as operating on the wrong patient or the wrong limb. The principal dangers encountered by American patients are much more insidious and therefore even more dangerous.

When a surgeon selects and performs one of several available surgical procedures, there are four possible outcomes for the patient:

1. The right operation performed well
2. The right operation performed badly
3. The wrong operation performed well
4. The wrong operation performed badly

In only one case (the right operation performed well) will the patient have the best result. Even if the surgical procedure chosen for a given condition is the correct one, a patient may be subjected to dangerous complications if the technical performance is inadequate.

On the other hand, if the wrong surgical procedure is chosen, it really doesn't matter how much technical skill goes into the performance: The patient will still not get well. The worst of all possible worlds, of course, is to have the wrong operation done poorly. Thus, in three ways out of four it's possible for the surgeon to err and for your surgery to be unsuccessful. All of these examples are errors of commission—choosing the wrong operation or performing it poorly. Many such errors may be hidden—for example, persistent symptoms after surgery may be attributed to continuation of the underlying disease process, whereas in reality they were caused by inadequate operative technique—and not all are as obvious as operating on the wrong patient.

In addition to the errors of commission, however, there are almost limitless possibilities for errors of omission. These are even less obvious and more difficult to detect than errors of commission. Failure to correctly diagnose and operate on a perforated ulcer by mistaking it for intestinal flu, or neglecting to examine the breasts of a patient who is later found to have breast cancer, are but two examples of errors of omission.

In short, there are many opportunities for a surgeon to err; the success of your operation depends to a large part on everything being done correctly.

Your risk from surgery can be considerably improved by avoiding the bad surgeons. If you can do just that, you can significantly improve your chances of staying alive and having a successful surgical procedure. Practically speaking, how can this be done? And even if you could avoid the bad surgeons, would you be satisfied with a mediocre surgeon? Don't you want the best?

One of the purposes of this book is to guide you in your selection of a surgeon. By giving you practical information on what to expect and what to look for, this book will help you to recognize a good surgeon and, if necessary, to find that surgeon yourself.

Unfortunately, finding a good surgeon is not all you have to worry about. Many professionals and support personnel must come together to forge a positive result. Physicians, surgeons, anesthesiologists, nurses, technicians, therapists, hospital administrators, and support personnel all work in concert to achieve one goal: your recovery. So although the surgeon plays a very important role in your surgical experience, the actions of the others also materially affect the outcome. When you finish this book, you will understand how each of these professionals fits into the surgical experience and what is the scope of their individual responsibilities. Finally, in addition to learning how to interact with your doctors and to play an active, informed role in your operation and recovery, you'll be better able to avoid needless surgery.

1

AN OVERVIEW OF SURGERY

Surgery, from the Latin word *chirurgia* (in turn from the Greek, *cheir,* hand, and *ergon,* work), literally means handiwork. Simply put, it's the treatment of disease by use of the hand. Yet the discipline of surgery would be useless if it weren't for the innate ability of human tissue to heal. Imagine for a moment: Without that healing ability, the slightest injury or disease would result, at the very least, in a lifelong defect.

HISTORY

Despite the intrinsic biological advantage afforded by healing, the development of surgery as a useful method of treatment was hindered throughout history by the presence of two major limitations:

- Pain (designed for the protection of the organism)
- Infection, the ancient nemesis of surgery, with its attendant high mortality rate

Nonetheless, surgery has been practiced for thousands of years. Physical evidence of surgical procedures actually precedes recorded history. Archaeologists have found examples of healed fractures in prehistoric human bones, suggesting setting and splinting by primitive "orthopedists." Skulls from the Neolithic period (10,000–7,000 B.C.) have been found with sections surgically removed (trepanation), a forerunner of modern skull decompression for head injury.

The first recorded surgical procedures—the Edwin Smith Papyrus (1600 B.C.), in which the care of 48 patients with various traumatic wounds is described—came from ancient Egypt. Quality control for surgeons was strictly maintained in those times. Surgeons must have selected their patients very carefully, refusing all risky cases, since Babylonian law called for removal of the surgeon's right hand if a patient died. (By comparison, today's malpractice suits seem mere annoyances.)

Primarily because of pain and infection, the full development of surgery as a useful method for the treatment of disease was delayed for more than 3,000 years. For all practical purposes, ancient surgical operations were restricted to lesions near the surface of the body. By the time of the Middle Ages, surgery had fallen into the hands of magicians, spell-casters, charlatans, and poorly educated but well-meaning practitioners. These surgical practitioners learned their limited craft in groups known as guilds, the forerunners of modern trade unions. The guilds were mutually exclusive trade schools composed of individuals with similar professional interests. Since sharp tools were required by barbers as well as surgeons, the graduates of this particular guild performed both functions interchangeably. They were known as barber-surgeons. In fact, the red stripes on a barber pole actually represent the ancient advertisement for bloodletting. Barber-surgeons were referred to as Mister, in order to further distance them from the "real" doctors, graduates of universities. As a result of this tradition, English surgeons even today are called Mister rather than Doctor. Itinerant graduates of this guild roamed Europe with occasional success, but more often wreaking havoc upon a helpless populace who had few alternatives. In the hands of such uninformed, undisciplined, and often unsavory practitioners, surgery fell into widespread disrepute. The term *barber-surgeon* remained an epithet for centuries.

With the discovery of ether as a general anesthetic agent by Crawford Long of Georgia in 1842, a major limitation was removed from the future development of surgery. No longer was it necessary for surgeons to operate with unsafe haste so as to reduce the magnitude and duration of pain. Operations could now be performed even inside the body.

The second landmark development in the history of surgery was the discovery by Louis Pasteur in 1865 that bacteria were the cause of surgical infections. It remained for Joseph Lister in Scotland to describe antiseptic surgery in 1867. By using a spray of carbolic acid on surgical instruments, the surgeons' hands, and surgical wounds, infection rates were substantially reduced.

But the twentieth century has witnessed the greatest

strides in medical and surgical progress. New and better operative procedures are being developed and studied with increasing frequency. Today we live in an era of dynamic change in surgical techniques in which everyone can benefit.

WHAT DOES SURGERY DO?

Surgery uses mechanical means to correct defects in body tissues caused by disease or injury. It can be described as concerned with four R's:

1. Resection: removal of diseased tissue (e.g., cancer surgery)
2. Restoration: using local tissues in the affected area to restore structure (e.g., hernia repair)
3. Reconstruction: using other tissues or tissue substitutes to reestablish function (e.g., blood-vessel surgery)
4. Replacement: substitution of new tissues for old (e.g., kidney transplantation)

Exactly how these general mechanical procedures are applied in specific situations is the technical craft of surgery. Mastering the craft requires intensive training and a lifelong commitment to continuing surgical education.

WHERE IS SURGERY PERFORMED?

Surgery may be performed in a hospital setting (so-called inpatient surgery), since at least one night is spent in the hospital for recovery. Because surgical operations requiring overnight hospitalization are usually the more complex procedures, this type of surgery is often called "major surgery." Less complex operations, which can be performed without the need for overnight hospitalization, are known as outpatient surgery and are sometimes considered "minor surgery." But the terms *major* and *minor surgery* have less meaning today, as increasingly more complex surgical procedures are being done in the outpatient setting.

Even surgical procedures that require general anesthesia are now being done as outpatient surgery. This type of surgery is known as ambulatory surgery, or A.M. surgery, since the patient walks into surgery in the morning, walks out in the afternoon, and recovers at home. Some relatively simple procedures are even performed in a doctor's office. Where your particular operation should be done is covered more fully in Chapter 12.

WHO DOES WHAT SURGERY?

One hundred years ago, most surgical procedures were performed by every surgeon, but the increasing complexity of surgical science and technology has led more and more to specialization. It's no longer possible—if it ever was—for any surgeon to remain current and highly qualified in all fields of surgery. Accordingly, surgeons today tend to specialize.

Basic training in general surgery still covers a wide range of knowledge and techniques in the treatment of problems of the head and neck; breast, abdomen, and extremities; and of the gastrointestinal, vascular, and endocrine systems. Some surgeons have special qualifications in the management of disorders of the blood vessels (vascular surgery); the care of infants and children (pediatric surgery); or in the treatment of critically ill patients in emergency departments or in intensive care, trauma, or burn units (surgical critical care). Other surgical specialties include colon and rectal surgery for the treatment of diseases of the intestinal tract, rectum, and anus; neurological surgery, dealing with disorders of the brain and nervous system; orthopedic surgery for the treatment of skeletal bones, muscles, and joints; otolaryngology, for the treatment of disorders of the head and neck, including the ears, nose, and throat; plastic surgery, focusing on cosmetic and reconstructive procedures; and thoracic surgery, concerned with the organs within the chest cavity, including the lungs, heart, and esophagus.

In addition, doctors in other specialties are often trained to perform surgery in their particular areas of expertise. These include dermatologists, obstetrician/gynecologists, ophthalmologists ("eye doctors"), and urologists.

Surgeons are actually permitted to do any type of surgery in which they have demonstrated competence, so it's important that you determine the qualifications and abilities of your proposed surgeon.

WHEN SHOULD YOU CONSIDER SURGERY?

All surgery has inherent risks. Naturally, if there are simpler, less risky ways to accomplish the desired result, they should be tried first. Although there are exceptions to this general rule, for example, for some forms of cancer and severe injuries, surgery should rarely be offered to patients before nonsurgical measures—medications, bed rest, or physical therapy—have been tried and failed, or at least been considered. For that reason, surgery is called a referral specialty, in which patients are usually referred by primary-care physicians after medical treatment has failed or been deemed inappropriate.

An important corollary to this principle is that patients are often sent to a surgeon late in the course of their disease. Such delays in referral and the advanced or complicated nature of conditions requiring surgery make a comparison of medical and surgical treatments for some diseases difficult, if not impossible.

In general, whenever medical and surgical treatments for a given condition offer comparable results, you should opt for the medical treatment first. This is why you should make sure that your doctors thoroughly explain all treatment options to you. If you remain undecided as to which treatment to choose, ask for more information. It is your right (and your responsibility) to understand everything that is being proposed about your treatment.

In your first visit with a prospective surgeon, ask just how your operation will be performed. It is probably not necessary for you to learn all the countless details, but a patient who wants to know exactly what the surgeon plans to do at the time of surgery, what equipment will be used, and how the operation is supposed to work can begin to develop a trusting relationship with the surgeon. But you may have to ask. It's amazing how many people have surgery without the slightest idea of what the surgeon did, or even which organ was affected! Ask your surgeon to show you on a diagram or model what he or she plans to do.

If you encounter any reluctance in helping you understand how your operation will be conducted, or if your surgeon is "too busy" to explain the operation to you, you may be dealing with someone who will be too busy to take care of you after the operation. Should you encounter such behavior, consider changing surgeons. You can ask your personal physician to recommend another surgeon or, if you wish, you can find one yourself (see Chapter 6).

2

"YOU NEED AN OPERATION"

It's only natural to want to avoid something unpleasant; the more unpleasant a situation is, the less you want to have anything to do with it. Perhaps this is why, when most people are faced with the prospect of surgery for themselves or for those closest to them, they prefer to delegate all such decisions to others and resign themselves to fate. They might even rationalize transferring such decisions to "those more qualified to make them." But abdicating responsibility for your health and well-being may have dangerous consequences.

For you to play a significant role in your surgical experience, it's important for you to overcome a considerable amount of anxiety. What do you really know about surgery in general? Or, for that matter, surgeons in particular? Do you really need this operation? Can you really trust someone you don't know with your life and well-being, even if the surgeon has been highly recommended? What are your chances of not making it? Or could you be disabled or have to live the rest of your life in pain?

"I'm Afraid the News Isn't Good . . ."

The past three months have been anything but fun. That gnawing pain in the top of your stomach has been getting slowly worse. At first, it was there for only a little while every few days. Now it seems to be there most of the time. Whenever you eat it gets worse, and now your back has begun to hurt. At first you hoped it would go away. Then you knew it wouldn't. What could it be? An ulcer? Gallbladder trouble? Cancer?

Finally, you make an appointment to see Mark; for years he's been more than just your family doctor, he's been your friend. When nothing showed up on routine tests, he suggested hospitalization. The past few days have been a blur of X rays, blood tests, and tubes placed in every orifice. Now Mark is standing at the foot of the bed holding an X ray. He isn't smiling. What is he going to say?

"I'm afraid the news isn't good. You've got a lump in your pancreas. It looks like a tumor."

What and where is your pancreas? A tumor! Does that mean cancer?

"Look here on the X ray. This is your pancreas, and this is the tumor. Can you see that?"

You see something, but you don't know what it is.

"There's a chance it could be malignant. If it is a malignancy, I think you'd be better off having the operation in a place where they do more of this kind of

work. I want you to see Ralph for a surgical consultation. He's the best surgeon at the General Hospital in Metropolis. He does this kind of work all the time, and I know you'll like him."

So it's serious! Mark didn't even mention the local surgeon. You've never been to Metropolis, and you've never heard of this doctor. But if Mark tells you the doctor is good, he must be. Still . . . this is serious. How can you tell if he's as good as Mark thinks? If you're going to put your life in his hands, you want to be sure. Should you get a second opinion? Would Mark be offended? You've never had an operation. What can surgery do anyway? Where do you turn if Mark can't answer your questions? You need help!

THE PSYCHOLOGY OF SURGERY

For most people, having an operation means entering an emotional twilight zone, full of anxiety and uncertainty. You're surrounded by people you don't know, in a place you've never been, about to undergo something you don't really understand. Small wonder that the prospect of surgery evokes some pretty frightening thoughts.

Anxiety is compounded when the proposed surgery is to be carried out under general anesthesia. Unspoken fears of being put to sleep and having things done to one's body while unconscious are common. Surgery differs from most other medical disciplines in that actual invasion of the patient's body occurs. The idea of having someone "plowing around" inside one's body is disturbing to many people. Finally, and most important, the prospect of surgery elicits the realistic fear of pain, and the insidious fear of death. Not many of us relish the thought of discomfort and pain, even if the pain is somewhat controlled. Few patients facing surgery have not imagined the possibility of their own death and the effect it would have on their loved ones.

To add to all this unpleasantness, the hospital environment often demands that you assume a passive and compliant role. You're told what to do, and you're expected to conform. Since most people don't know what's best for them in a surgical situation, submission seems the wisest course. Yet it can be very frightening to lose control of your destiny, especially when you lose it to a group of comparative strangers. Many people experience deep feelings of helplessness and frustration.

Often it's just such fears that cause you to delay seeking medical help, in the hope that your condition is only temporary and that it will improve by itself without treatment or surgery. The dynamic balance between hope and fear is immobilizing for many people and frequently causes delay in seeking help. Such procrastination often results in advanced and occasionally even incurable conditions. These same fears may also cause you to assume a passive role and prevent you from having any significant input into your surgical experience. Ironically, your failure to be included in the decision-making process may actually contribute to the one thing you want the least—a poor surgical outcome.

Illnesses that are well treated by medication alone are often regarded as comparatively minor, and in such cases patients often continue their daily lives with only temporary inconvenience. Conditions requiring surgery, on the other hand, tend to be regarded as more serious and capable of disrupting a person's current and future life. Furthermore, surgical treatment can be serious in itself. The combination of a serious disease and a serious treatment demands your full attention.

DEALING WITH FEAR

The prospect of surgery forces you to face the possibility of your own mortality, an unpleasant prospect at best. For many people, this is the first time they have seriously considered the possibility that they may die. Instead of suppressing these fears, you need to understand that it's normal to be afraid of surgery. Such fears do not reflect cowardice in any way, but are emotional evidence of a deep unconscious commitment to life. Patients who claim to have no fear of surgery either have unrealistic expectations of the safety and curative powers of surgery or they are subconsciously blocking reality.

In addition to general fears about surgery, certain surgical procedures may produce additional concerns and anxiety:

- Mastectomy raises complex psychological issues in addition to those evoked by the cancer's threat to life. In some cases, the operation can mutilate an organ that for many women is related to self-esteem and sexual expression. For these reasons, deep-seated emotions must be taken into account when planning breast surgery.
- Colostomy and ileostomy can also provoke psychological issues in patients, because they result in bowel contents draining directly into a bag on the surface of the skin. Fortunately, newer methods of collecting the intestinal contents have decreased

much of the unpleasantness associated with these procedures, and newer operations have reduced the necessity of resorting to them.

- Other surgical procedures such as coronary artery bypass and hysterectomy are often emotionally charged. Transplantation of kidneys and hearts can evoke emotional concerns in both donors and recipients. It's difficult for many people to imagine the impact of feeling another person's heart beating inside them or of knowing that someone else's kidney is keeping them alive.
- Finally, cosmetic surgery may produce considerable anxiety. This form of surgery differs from others in that the chief purpose is not correction of illness. The primary goals of cosmetic surgery are a gain in self-esteem and improvement in appearance and emotional well-being. Results from cosmetic surgery often reflect a delicate balance between a patient's emotional expectations and reality.

An appreciation that certain surgical procedures may be associated with emotional stress over and above the general anxieties produced by surgery is necessary for patients, their families, and surgeons.

Because they know very little about the surgical process, many people find themselves in a role of increasing dependency when faced with the prospect of surgery. It's far too easy for patients to delegate to the surgeon all responsibility for the critical decisions involved in their care, but doing so leads to maximum vulnerability for the patient. It is possible, however, to reach a middle ground, one where you can participate in much of the important decision-making and planning, thereby reducing your vulnerability.

At some point, your ability to control the surgical process will cease. This is when it becomes necessary for you to trust your surgeon to make the remaining decisions correctly. Indeed, trust is the cornerstone of the surgeon-patient relationship. A sensitive surgeon, skilled in the complexities of that relationship, will try to earn your confidence. If you're fortunate enough to have a surgeon who earns your trust, who you believe to be capable and caring, many of the normal fears and anxieties associated with surgery will diminish.

By placing your life in the surgeon's hands, you grant the ultimate trust possible between two persons. For precisely that reason, the bond between patient and surgeon is often intense. Patients often ascribe impossibly idealistic attributes to their surgeons—infallibility, supreme virtuosity—perhaps to reaffirm that their trust has not been misplaced. Being convinced that your surgeon is the best makes it easier for you to delegate responsibility and grant trust. But not everyone's surgeon can be the best. There are not enough of those to go around.

Yet you can ascertain whether your surgeon is capable of performing the operation you need, and you can select the surgeon you believe is best for the procedure you require. When you take an active role in choosing your surgeon, you can more easily place your trust in that person.

What can you do about overcoming the natural fears of surgery? Perhaps the best thing you can do is realize that fears can be both rational and irrational. Unfortunately, the rational ones—such as the fear of death or disability—are inevitable with the prospect of surgery. Irrational fears—such as a sense of impending doom—can be immobilizing and terrifying. But learning as much as you can about surgery in general, your operation in particular, and the surgeon who will perform it will help to minimize many of the fears that may arise.

3

SURVIVAL AND SUCCESS

For most people, the two most important questions about surgery are: Am I going to live through the operation? and, If I do survive, will I be better? In other words, Doc, what are my chances?

Your chances are remarkably good. If we could lump all surgical procedures together, your chances of making it through would be considerably better than 95 out of 100. Survival from any individual operation depends on numerous variables and may be 10 to 100 times better than this average figure, or 10 to 100 times worse.

It could be said, however, that for the 5 out of 100 who do not survive, the odds were pretty bad. Since no single person is "average" regardless of the proposed operation, each patient must face some degree of risk.

HOW SUCCESSFUL IS SURGERY?

Although we do not have overall cure figures for every possible surgical procedure, if they were known, they would certainly be less than the 95 percent chance of survival. Simply put, your chances of surviving surgery are better than your chances of being cured. How much better depends on the disease or condition being treated, on your own physical and emotional makeup, and the surgical team's performance.

For some conditions, such as gallstones, surgery is 85 percent successful; for others, such as severe trauma, your chances for cure may be little better than 50/50. Even worse are those conditions, such as internal malignancies, for which surgery is usually unsuccessful but in which surgery offers the only chance. The nature and severity of the underlying disease or condition are greater determinants for cure than for survival.

Can you ever be certain that you will survive and benefit from surgery? Absolute certainty doesn't exist in medicine, and guarantees are therefore unreliable. All diseases, all patients, all hospitals, and all doctors are not the same, so common sense tells us that all results will not be the same. Any number of factors can influence the outcome of any surgical procedure. The interplay of those factors will raise or lower your chances of a good result.

The Complexity of the Condition

In general, the risks of surgery rise and the benefits of surgery fall as the underlying condition becomes complicated. A good example of this is removal of the appendix for acute appendicitis. If the appendix has not ruptured, the mortality risk for an appendectomy is approximately 1 in 3,000. But if the appendix has burst, spreading infection inside the abdomen, the death rate after surgery can be as high as 3 in 100. Although both rates are quite low, there's a hundredfold increase in mortality risk when the appendix ruptures and the condition becomes complicated. Obviously, an operation performed before complications develop carries a lower risk of mortality and a greater chance for a favorable outcome.

The Type of Lesion Certain diseases and conditions, by their very nature, are more difficult to treat surgically than others. That open-heart surgery is more formidable than hernia repair is obvious. The surgical treatment of localized infections (abscesses) is more likely to be successful than spinal fusion, cataract surgery is usually more successful than sinus surgery, and so forth. There's a hierarchy of severity for surgical diseases and conditions which, even in the absence of other contributing factors, strongly affects results.

Anatomic Location Much has to do with the technical difficulty of surgery in the specific organ. The more vital the organ operated on, the more difficult the surgery. Brain, liver, pancreas, and heart surgery present technical challenges that require expert surgeons. Usually, if the operation is technically difficult for the surgeon, it will be difficult for the patient as well. A difficult operation can be a technical success yet fail miserably as far as results are concerned. And after all, the patient is concerned only with results.

Timing of Surgery The timing of an operation is also very important. Excessive delay often permits the underlying condition to advance in severity. The more severe the condition, the worse the chances for a good outcome. Similarly, an operation performed as an emergency may have significantly poorer results than the same operation performed "electively," at a time mutually selected by the patient and the surgeon. An operation performed before complications develop carries a lower risk of mortality and a greater chance for a favorable result.

Many other factors, such as the skill of the surgeon, the capability of the anesthesiologist, and the scope of the hospital resources, also affect survival and success and are discussed in subsequent chapters.

Patient Factors

The overall condition of the patient prior to surgery is an important determinant of surgical risk. The same operation performed on a healthy athlete and on a debilitated patient with heart or lung disease usually does not yield the same results. The existence of other conditions or diseases, such as kidney disease, diabetes, malnutrition, or liver disease, increases the risk of mortality and poor results from surgery. Personal habits such as smoking or excessive alcohol intake may also have a negative impact on your chances.

Your willingness to comply with your surgeon's directions is often a deciding factor in determining results from surgery. For example, certain potentially fatal complications of surgery, such as pulmonary emboli (blood clots in the lungs) or pneumonia, can often be prevented if a patient gets out of bed and begins to move about very soon after surgery. But walking after major surgery is often uncomfortable, so compliance with the surgeon's advice may take a considerable effort from a patient who is feeling weak and shaky.

The first few days after major surgery are the most critical. In the immediate postoperative period, your mental attitude goes a long way toward determining the quality of your recovery and the length of your hospitalization. Patients who are determined to get well after surgery usually do. Such people "refuse to be sick" and try to get back to normal almost immediately. Other patients adopt a more passive or self-protecting approach, letting others tend to their needs. Their recovery is likely to proceed more slowly and may be hindered by emotional difficulties.

Many physicians and surgeons have observed that patients with a positive, confident attitude tolerate surgery better than those who have a more negative, worrying outlook. Even though we don't fully understand the psychosomatic mechanisms involved, many surgeons are convinced that a patient's mental attitude significantly affects his or her physical response to surgery. We know that the brain regulates many of the body's physical defenses against injury and infection. If surgery can be regarded as "controlled injury," it seems likely that some connection can be made between mental attitude and physical recovery. Future research may well establish a neurohormonal link to account for these clinical observations. But regardless of the mechanisms involved, you can really help yourself by leaving business, marital, financial, and other worries at home when you undergo surgery so you can concentrate on getting well.

4

EXPECTATIONS

Suppose your doctor has recommended surgery for your problem. Exactly what should you expect? Are your expectations reasonable? If not, which of your hopes are realistic and which are not? Patients with unrealistic expectations are bound to be disappointed.

WHAT SHOULD YOU EXPECT FROM YOUR SURGEON?

You have a right to expect your surgeon to be a complete doctor. It's easy to place too much emphasis on technical skill as the outstanding attribute of a surgeon. But in actual fact, surgical judgment is even more important. Certainly a surgeon must have the motor skills necessary for the technical performance of an operation, but a good surgeon is more than a mere "tissue technician." Although many people (and unfortunately even some surgeons) see surgery only as the dramatic episode that takes place in the operating room, surgery is much more than just the operation itself.

Properly preparing a patient for surgery and taking care of the patient after surgery are as important as the actual operation. Surgery involves knowing when (and when not) to operate, how to put the patient in the best shape to tolerate surgery, which operation to choose, and what is needed for recovery after surgery. All of this is in addition to being able to perform the operation itself. To operate on a patient and leave the pre- and postoperative care entirely to someone else restricts surgery to a mere technical exercise and often indicates a lack of respect and little concern for the patient as a person. Some might even consider it unethical. You should expect your surgeon to be involved in your care before and after surgery.

Of course, no single doctor can know everything. Even the best-intentioned and best-trained surgeon encounters problems for which specialized advice should be sought. Good surgeons are not afraid to ask for consultations with other physicians. The important point is this: Your surgeon should remain in control of your case throughout your hospital course and should not delegate your care to someone else. Although you may also be seen by other doctors—your primary-care doctor or another surgeon covering for your surgeon—the operating surgeon knows best what to expect from this surgery, what complications can arise, and how to diagnose and treat them. If your surgeon is too busy to see you before surgery, and not available to take care of you after your operation, look for one who has more interest in you as a human being and not as just another operation.

You have a right to expect your surgeon to recognize his or her personal limitations. No surgeon is capable of performing all possible operations equally well, and some surgeons are better equipped than others for a particular procedure. You have a right to know how much experience your surgeon has had with your proposed operation and what results were achieved. If you find a surgeon who doesn't hesitate to put your interests first and who refers you to a colleague who is better able to perform the operation you need, remember that surgeon's name. If you should need less complicated surgery in the future, you will have found a caring surgeon with integrity.

You have a right to expect your surgeon to take pride in his or her work. Most surgeons do, and they suffer emotionally when results are not as good as they expect. This commitment to excellence is bred into surgical trainees early on and should become an integral part of each surgeon's attitude. You can often get a sense of this commitment during your initial discussions. It's a necessary quality of a good surgeon. Look for it!

INFORMED CONSENT

You have a right to expect a full explanation of your condition, how surgery will affect it, whether there are good alternatives to surgery, and what risks or complications are associated with the operation. All of these considerations are part of the process of "informed consent," a discussion with your surgeon of why the surgery is recommended, which operation is proposed, what complications can occur, and what you can expect if the operation is a success. This discussion should help you crystallize your expectations, and give you an opportunity to decline the surgery as well.

This discussion is extremely important. Pay close attention, and don't tune it out. If you agree to surgery after everything has been explained to you, you will be sharing in the responsibility for the decision to operate. Be leery of the surgeon who doesn't have enough time to discuss these things with you.

You can and should continue to ask questions until you understand exactly what is being proposed and why. You should be given enough information to make a reasonable decision to accept or reject surgery. Your doctors are only offering their opinion, which you may or may not choose to accept. Ultimately, it's your decision whether or not to have surgery. Make sure you get enough information to make that decision intelligently.

The informed-consent discussion gives you a chance to judge what kind of person your surgeon is. Are you satisfied with the answers you get? Does the doctor communicate patience and compassion, sincerity and warmth? Or can you be comfortable dealing with a surgeon who is detached and businesslike, focused and objective?

Deciding to recommend surgical intervention in any disease process always requires careful consideration. Surgical treatment becomes an option only after other forms of therapy have failed or are ruled out. Even then, surgery may not offer an advantage over no treatment at all. What will happen if nothing is done? The "zero-treatment option" should always be part of any discussion of treatment choices.

It is your right (and your responsibility) to accept or reject the proposed operation. The informed-consent discussion should provide you with all the information you need to make that decision.

WHAT RESULTS CAN YOU EXPECT?

Perfect results from surgery are more likely due to a series of fortunate coincidences than just to the skill of the surgeon. If your diagnosis is correct, if surgery is an accepted and successful treatment for that diagnosis, if the operation is properly chosen and performed, and if there are no complications, you should expect to be improved, if not completely well.

An intimate knowledge of your condition, combined with an understanding of the values and risks of the proposed surgery, gives your surgeon the ability to predict what result you may reasonably expect. But so many factors go into determining results from surgery that unexpected developments may alter even the most circumspect predictions.

Many important elements of a surgical experience are beyond the direct control of the surgeon: the quality of anesthesia, laboratory reliability, hospital regulations and facilities management, to name just a few. Each of these can significantly affect the results of surgery. We can say what results will follow surgery in 100 patients with your condition: A certain percentage will be cured, a certain percentage improved, some unchanged, and a few worse. What we don't know is where you, as an individual, will fit into those statistical norms.

Predicting the outcome for an individual patient is difficult even under the best conditions. It's wise to regard your surgeon's prediction of results as a guideline rather than a promise. There can be no guarantees where surgery is concerned. Patients should not expect them, and ethical surgeons won't give them to you. Furthermore, remember that other forms of medical treatment may have failed before surgery was ever considered, and if your condition could have been treated by easier means, it would have been. Seen in this light, surgery is often a last resort, and under these circumstances, perfection should never be promised or expected.

Pain is a necessary accompaniment of most types of surgery. Although pain can be completely controlled by anesthesia during surgery, complete pain control after the operation is undesirable. Total abolition of pain often results in stupor, which in turn leads to shallow breathing and risk of pneumonia or immobility and risk of fatal lung clots. For these and other reasons, postoperative analgesics (pain medications) are designed to minimize pain, not to eliminate it entirely. Fortunately, improvements in postoperative pain control have markedly reduced the discomfort associated with surgery (see Chapter 10). Moreover, even the pain of major surgery decreases markedly by the second or third postoperative day, and most people tolerate the small amount of discomfort necessary to prevent complications.

In the absence of surgical infection or bleeding, it's remarkable how fast the body recovers from surgical injury. Although individual rates of recovery do vary, the average hospital stay for major surgery is now less than six days. If you've had major surgery, you probably won't be 100 percent back to normal in a week or even longer. Your surgeon can give you guidelines for gradually resuming normal activities. In general, you should go back to work when you think you're able, resting even longer if your job requires physical exertion or if you find yourself tiring easily.

What about the scar? Will it be small, faint, and barely visible, or will it be genuinely disfiguring? In the absence of infection, bleeding, or a tendency to form thick scars (keloids), most surgical scars are acceptable. If the incision is in a particularly noticeable place, or if you have any reason for wanting a finer scar than usual, be sure to discuss it with your surgeon. There are special techniques that can sometimes be used to minimize a scar, but these techniques may require a plastic surgeon, may be difficult to perform, and may be too time-consuming to be used in areas that are not commonly exposed. Your surgeon may be able to comply with your request.

5

HOW SURGEONS ARE MADE

Before one can become a surgeon, one must first become a doctor of medicine. Each year more than 30,000 students apply for approximately 12,000 places in America's 127 medical schools. Each applicant must demonstrate a high level of undergraduate scholarship, and few acceptances are given to students with a grade point average below 3.5 (out of a possible 4.0). Courses in biology, chemistry, and physics are usually required for a major in premed, in addition to a range of liberal arts courses, such as English, mathematics, philosophy, psychology, and foreign languages.

Medical school applicants must take an overall test of information called the Medical College Admissions Test (MCAT). Well-qualified applicants, with high scores and persuasive recommendations from college advisers and deans, are invited for interviews by medical school admissions offices. Each student may interview for as many medical schools as offer invitations.

Personal interviews give a school's admissions committee an opportunity to evaluate motivation and compassion, along with other qualities considered desirable, such as emotional stability, honesty, and affability. The student may attend any school offering an acceptance.

FOREIGN MEDICAL SCHOOLS

Students not accepted by an American medical school may attend foreign medical schools if they wish. Many of these accept any and all applicants, regardless of qualifications. Only a few have entry criteria as stringent as those for American schools. Unfortunately, there is often little regulation of course content or quality in foreign medical schools. (In contrast, there are several supervisory agencies that monitor and regulate the quality of American medical schools, thus directly maintaining a high quality of graduates.) Also, there is often little hands-on experience for students, and a lack of such direct patient contact markedly limits the ability of these students to perform when confronted with real people and real problems. Book learning is of course important, but the knowledge gained from books must be applied to patients through practical experience. For these and other reasons, foreign medical graduates (FMGs) are often at a severe disadvantage when compared to graduates of American medical schools. Although there are many exceptions to this generalization, you might wish to keep it in mind when evaluating surgeons.

CURRICULUM

The American medical school curriculum usually consists of two years of classroom and laboratory work in basic sciences (anatomy, biochemistry, physiology, microbiology, pharmacology, and pathology), followed by two years of active involvement in patient care in clinical settings. Patients are seen by students under the supervision of senior doctors, usually in a hospital affiliated with the medical school or the parent university. After completing medical school and successfully passing two tests given to each American medical student (Steps I and II of the U.S. Medical Licensing Examinations—USMLE), the student is granted the diploma of Doctor of Medicine (M.D.).

LICENSING

Before the graduate can go into practice, however, additional postgraduate, or residency, training is required. Since a doctor cannot practice medicine in the United States without a state license, individual states are free to set additional requirements as qualifications for licensure, such as the length of residency training or a state licensing examination. At least one year of postgraduate hospital training is required before the physician-to-be is permitted to take a third qualifying examination, either the USMLE

Part III or the examination given by the Federation of State Medical Licensing Boards (FLEX). Only then is the novice doctor permitted to apply for an unrestricted license to practice medicine.

SURGICAL RESIDENCY

In the past, the first year of training after medical school graduation was called "internship" and the subsequent years were called "residency." Now, all postgraduate trainees are known as residents, differentiated by the number of years out of medical school: postgraduate-year-one resident (PGY 1), postgraduate-year-two resident (PGY 2), and so forth. The length of a surgical residency varies with the surgical specialty, from five to eight years, and some even longer.

During this time of residency, a fledgling surgeon learns how to apply the knowledge and crafts of surgery to the care of patients. This is accomplished through a process of graded responsibility. In the initial years of surgical residency, the emphasis is placed on preoperative and postoperative care rather than the acquisition of specialized operative techniques. In these early years, the surgical resident is the most junior member of the surgical team, carrying out the less complex tasks of caring for surgical patients: drawing blood, inserting tubes, changing dressings, and writing medical orders (scut work). In addition, the resident surgeon goes to the operative suite as a second or third assistant to the responsible surgeon. These tasks can be extremely time consuming. A workday of 18 to 20 hours and 90- to 120-hour weeks are common. There is little free time. Most surgical programs require the resident to spend every second or third night in the hospital.

Residents get on-the-job training in operating rooms, on wards, and at the bedside as well as in classrooms, laboratories, and the library. Textbooks, professional journals, videotapes, and interactive computer programs may be used as well. Progress (or the lack of it) is monitored by "attendings," experienced surgeons who supervise and evaluate the care given to patients by the residents. Attendings usually have university appointments and may also be full- or part-time employees of the medical school or hospital. They take direct responsibility for the care residents provide to the patients.

Each year the resident takes a national exam, the American Board of Surgery In-Training Examination (ABSITE), designed to evaluate basic knowledge and clinical skills. Individuals are compared to national averages, and specific areas of deficiency are noted. If satisfactory progress is made in basic surgical knowledge and clinical skills, the resident advances to the next higher level, from PGY 1 to PGY 2, for example.

During the early years of surgical training, all surgical residents are enrolled in a general surgical training program, in which they are exposed to all types of surgery: abdominal; breast; cardiac and thoracic (chest); ear, nose, and throat; gynecological; orthopedic; transplantation; urological; pediatric; and plastic surgery, as well as anesthesia and critical care. The residents thus experience many brief periods (usually two to four months) of highly concentrated training in many types of surgery.

After the first or second year of general surgical training, the resident must decide whether to continue in general surgery or to branch out into a surgical subspecialty, such as otolaryngology, neurosurgery, or orthopedics. Residents who wish to remain in general surgery must complete a minimum of five years of training. Many opt for an additional year or two of investigation in a research laboratory. Residents interested in pediatric surgery, colon and rectal surgery, or thoracic surgery must complete the five-year general surgery program before going on to the more specialized training programs. As residents progress through training, they are gradually given more responsibility in the operating room.

Although the attending surgeon "assists" the resident, in fact, it is the attending who controls the operation, making crucial decisions about how the procedure is to be performed. The attending often performs the most difficult parts of the operation and is always ready to take over from the resident if any problem arises. With the passage of time, as residents become more and more proficient in surgical techniques, they are given more control over the actual performance of the operation and they in turn supervise the work of more-junior residents.

At the end of the formal training period, surgical residents must be certified by the chief of the surgical department in which they have been trained. Such certification means that the resident has satisfactorily completed all the required elements of surgical training. Residents must submit a list of all the different operations they have performed during residency. This list, along with the chairperson's recommendation as to the character and ethics of the resident, is sent to the American Board of Surgery, the national certifying agency.

At this point, the recent graduate of an approved surgical residency training program is said to be board eligible and is permitted to apply to the specific surgical board for certification. Not everyone who trains in surgery becomes board eligible. Only training programs that have been approved by an independent agency are permitted to send their graduates for certification. Being board eligible is the minimum standard of excellence for surgeons.

To receive board certification from a specific subspecialty board, another examination is required. These written and oral examinations cover the theory and practice of each surgical specialty. They are rigorous tests that measure intellectual and clinical skills.

Not everyone who is board eligible becomes board certified. Approximately a third of board eligible surgeons fail the examinations necessary to gain certification.

The surgeon who is board certified in a specialty has come a long way. The time spent in education is staggering: 12 years of primary and high school, 4 years of college, 4 years of medical school, and 5 to 8 years of surgical residency. Many newly qualified surgeons are over 30 years old before beginning their own practice and have been in school for 24 of those 30-odd years.

6

CHOOSING A SURGEON

The decision to engage a particular surgeon is one of the most important decisions you will ever make. Your well-being, even your life, may be at risk. You can have confidence in that decision if you know what to look for. Armed with the information in this chapter, you can actively cooperate with your family doctor in choosing the right person to perform your operation.

Don't hesitate to take some control. It may require a slight change in your attitude, but you stand to gain a lot. Don't worry about offending anyone by wanting to participate in these decisions. Your family doctor should not be upset if you raise questions about his or her recommendations. And a prospective surgeon should not be offended if you ask questions in the process of making your decision.

THE SURGICAL REFERRAL

Most patients arrive in a particular surgeon's office as the result of a referral: The family doctor or a medical specialist has made the recommendation. If you get there by any other means, be careful! Accepting even well-intentioned medical advice from a friend or acquaintance can be dangerous. Choosing a prominent surgeon on the basis of reputation or because he or she has appeared in advertisements or on a talk show can be equally risky. Hospitals, specialty clinics, and groups of doctors increasingly tout their services in print and on the air, but cautious consumers should regard such advertising claims with skepticism.

Ideally, the recommendation should be made solely on the basis of merit. But referral decisions are often influenced by social or economic considerations. Family ties, school affiliations, social connections, or even personal compatibility can also play a part. That's not necessarily bad: If a surgeon has provided good service to the referring physician's patients with good results in the past, it's likely that a referral pattern will be established. But—and this is a very large "but"—that does not necessarily mean that that surgeon will be successful in your case. No two cases are exactly alike.

Changes in our health-care system have introduced new forms of referral that sometimes may compromise what freedom of choice physicians or patients have in choosing a surgeon. Prepaid health insurance plans often limit your choice to a panel of previously approved surgeons. A controlling goal of such plans (HMOs, PPOs, IPAs, etc.) is to reduce health-care expenses. For a surgeon to become approved by a given plan may involve little more than a willingness to reduce fees. Primary-care physicians who are employed by a prepaid health plan are usually required to refer patients only to surgeons within the same plan. In that situation, the primary-care physician (the gatekeeper) is not necessarily a guarantor of excellence, a connoisseur selecting the best from a wide range of possibilities; he or she may be merely an agent or broker choosing from a previously limited slate of available candidates. Patients may be at risk under such a system, since neither they nor their primary-care physician has free choice and surgical competence is not assured.

The choice of having the surgery at all may be limited. Some HMOs give primary-care doctors a "capitation" payment based on the number of patients who sign up for them. That payment is calculated to cover all the expected costs of treating those patients over a given period. Doctors must make sure that the costs of care don't exceed their capitation payments, so whereas a capitation payment is designed to eliminate incentives to overtreat, it can also create incentives to undertreat, particularly with regard to expensive specialty care, such as surgery.

What can the prospective surgical patient do about this? If your condition is a true emergency, the time available is limited and you will often be forced to accept whoever is recommended. As an alternative in an emergency situation, you usually won't go far wrong by going to the best hospital you know of and taking potluck with the surgeon on call. But it's also possible to prepare for the possibility of emergency surgery by gathering information in advance, when no urgency exists. In more relaxed situations, when you have enough time to make decisions, you need to know the right questions to ask.

HOW TO FIND A GOOD SURGEON

Of the 25 million operations performed in the United States in 1993, it has been estimated that as many as one third were performed by individuals who were not board certified. Today, of the more than 100,000 physicians practicing surgery of all types in the United States, more than one third (36 percent) are not board certified in any area of surgery.

If you need surgery, unless you're very careful, your chances are almost one in three of being operated on by a person who has failed either to complete an approved and lengthy residency or to pass the rigorous examinations required for board certification.

The obvious solution to this disparity in surgical competence would be for hospitals to restrict operating privileges exclusively to surgeons with board certification. Legal issues, such as restraint of trade or freedom of access, often surface when attempts are made to restrict hospital surgical privileges to board certified surgeons. In some states, merely graduating from medical school and spending an additional year in a general internship are all one needs to get a license to practice "medicine and surgery." But whereas organized medicine cannot restrict surgical privileges to board certified surgeons, you can. If all patients would demand board certification as a priority in their choice of a surgeon, the level of surgical competence in this country would be substantially improved.

These remarks should not be taken to mean that a surgeon without board certification can never be trusted to perform operations safely and well for some conditions. Many can and do perform competently. Similarly, board certification is not an absolute guarantee of surgical competence. The bottom line is this: Your chances of finding a competent surgeon are significantly higher when you demand board certification as the minimum qualification you will accept. Here, then, is the first question to ask a recommended surgeon:

- ***"Are you board certified in your surgical specialty?"***

Don't be embarrassed to ask this question. Those who are board certified won't mind telling you: They're justifiably proud of it. But if you're uncomfortable asking such a question, you can consult the *Directory of Medical Specialists,* usually available at local libraries. (You can obtain a copy by writing to Macmillan, Inc., 3002 Glenview Road, Wilmette, IL 60091.)

Is board certification enough to ensure surgical competence? Yes and no. Yes, if you have a common condition for which surgery is usually straightforward and successful (Tier I and Tier II procedures—see Chapter 9). If your problem is a hernia, breast lump, gallstones, or similar common problems, you can rest assured that most board certified surgeons are competent to do the job.

But if your condition is complex (Tier III procedures), rare, or made complicated by the presence of other diseases such as heart, lung, or kidney disease, board certification alone may not guarantee surgical competence. Under those conditions, you may need a more expert surgeon, one with experience in handling your kind of specialized case. One way of distinguishing more competent surgeons is membership in the American College of Surgeons.

The ACS was founded in 1913 "to improve the quality of care for surgical patients by elevating the standards of surgical education and practice." It is not a college in the usual sense, since it doesn't teach surgery to students. But it does sponsor continuing education and self-assessment courses for surgeons in practice as well as conducting nationwide programs to improve patient care. It is a professional society with more than 52,000 members from all fields of surgery and all parts of the country. To be elected to membership, a surgeon must be board certified and have practiced in a specific community for at least two years.

An important part of acceptance to membership in the ACS is peer review. Other surgeons from the same community judge the candidate's ethics, morals, and personality, as well as conducting on-site observations of the surgeon's competence. If accepted into membership, the candidate becomes a Fellow of the American College of Surgeons (FACS). Whereas board certification attests to a surgeon's knowledge and judgment, fellowship in the American College of Surgeons implies high moral and ethical standards as well. The second question to ask your prospective surgeon is:

- ***"Are you a Fellow of the American College of Surgeons?"***

Again, if you'd rather not ask so direct a question, see if your local library or a medical school library has a copy of the *American College of Surgeons Yearbook,* which lists alphabetically and by locality the names and addresses of all the Fellows of the College.

Alternatively, you can call the American College of Surgeons (312-664-4050), ask for the Communications Department, and inquire as to whether your surgeon is a member of the college. Upon request, the college will also send you a list of fellows from your geographic area.

But board certification and ACS membership may still not suffice. Those general credentials may not necessarily apply to your specific case. So you should ask a third question:

- ***"How many times have you performed the operation you are proposing for me?"***

If the answer is only a few times, you may wish to find a surgeon with more experience in that particular procedure.

Of course, it would also be good to know how well patients who have had this particular operation have done in the hands of your potential surgeon. You might want to ask question four:

- ***"How do your results compare with those of other surgeons?"***

For many common minor operations, being average will be perfectly acceptable. But it's important for you to consider the complexity of your condition in evaluating a response to this question.

Even in the best surgical hands and under the best surgical conditions, complications can occur. Although the chances that complications will develop in your case may be small, you should ask your surgeon about this possibility:

- ***"What sort of complications have you encountered with this operation, how often do they occur, and how do you manage them when they do occur?"***

As we mentioned in an earlier chapter, the facilities of the hospital are important, both before and after the operation. Good nursing care, up-to-date intensive care units, excellent support services, and readily available consultations can often mean the difference between living and dying. Hence, question six:

- *"Is the hospital equipped and staffed to manage a serious complication if it develops? Are consultations readily available?"*

Finally, you may wish to know how your surgeon is perceived by his or her colleagues and previous patients. That brings us to several other questions:

- *"Have you ever been the object of a professional peer review?"*
- *"Have you ever been censured?"*
- *"Have you ever been sued for malpractice? And if so, were you judged to be at fault?"*

Understandably, you may be uncomfortable asking such questions. Nevertheless, you do have a right to know, and if the answers are yes, you should be completely satisfied with the explanation offered or find another surgeon.

HOW TO FIND THE "BEST" SURGEON

Suppose your surgical condition is rare or complicated by other (co-morbid) conditions. In that case, it's even more important for you to find the appropriate surgeon. In rare or complicated surgical cases, having the right surgeon is often the key to survival. The surgeon who did such a wonderful job with your next-door neighbor's gallbladder operation may be completely out of his or her depth with your liver tumor. There's a hierarchy of difficulty in surgical cases; the more difficult the surgery, the more you need a highly specialized and experienced surgeon. If you question the difficulty of your condition, ask:

- ***"Does my condition need a surgeon who specializes in this sort of thing?"***

Suppose your condition does require such a surgeon. How can you find that expert, one who is truly above the average level of surgical competence? Experts are the surgeons to whom other surgeons send their most difficult and complicated cases. Good competent surgeons (those you have now learned to identify) know who the surgical experts are. So your last question should be:

- ***"Can you recommend an expert?"***

If you experience any difficulty with surgeon-to-surgeon referral, there are other approaches you can take. Often, surgical experts are superspecialists in certain organs or diseases, devoting most of their time to their sphere of interest, managing difficult cases referred by other surgeons. Many of these expert surgeons are connected with universities and medical schools, or with famous clinics. For every surgical disease, however great or small, there are surgeons who are considered to be experts in its management.

Surgical peer recognition takes many forms. Expert surgeons can often be recognized by their teaching commitments. They write chapters in major textbooks or articles in professional journals, and they teach other surgeons. Peer recognition is also evidenced by membership in the more than 80 prestigious national surgical societies. Each of the nine surgical specialties, such as general surgery, neurosurgery, and thoracic surgery, has one or more national societies to which surgeons may aspire as they become increasingly recognized as experts. Membership in one or more of these implies special qualifications in that discipline. The American Surgical Association is the oldest national surgical organization, with membership restricted to an elite group of nationally and internationally recognized experts from all fields of surgery. Although there can be no guarantees in surgery, you can be fairly certain that a surgeon who belongs to the American Surgical Association will bring to your case the highest level of knowledge, skill, and experience.

BEYOND THE OPERATING ROOM

Although time spent in the operating room is the most dramatic part of a surgeon's day, surgeons do many other things that are critical to surgical results. To be sure, the actual operative procedure is a necessary and important part of making the surgical patient better. The proper performance of cutting, clamping, and sewing tissue is what sets surgery apart from other medical disciplines. For that reason, good eye-hand coordination and highly developed motor skills are necessary attributes of a competent operating surgeon. Some truly gifted surgeons have developed these motor skills to a high degree and have become superb operative technicians.

But technical operative virtuosity is only part of being a good surgeon. The masterful placement of a clamp or the skillful introduction of a stitch can prevent fatal hemorrhage in the operating room. And the more technically proficient a surgeon is, the more likely it is that a patient will have a good result. But surgery is much more than that.

It is in the other aspects of surgery, the parts that have little to do with the drama of the operating room—in diagnosis, preoperative and postoperative care, even in knowing when not to operate—that surgical results are often decided and the truly competent surgeon shines.

Your surgeon must know how to get you into the best possible shape to withstand surgery, must choose the correct surgical operation for your condition from among numerous possibilities, and must be able to get you over the tissue damage and stress that accompany all forms of surgery. In determining the results from surgery, preoperative preparation and postoperative care are at least equal in importance to the actual operative procedure.

You may be reluctant to discuss qualifications when you first meet with the recommended surgeon, but remember what is at stake: Are you more concerned with the possibility of hurting the surgeon's feelings, or with actually improving your chances for staying alive and getting better? Truly good surgeons will not be offended by being asked to discuss their qualifications with you. Most surgeons are proud of their accomplishments, and they should welcome your active participation in the doctor-patient relationship.

7

SECOND THOUGHTS

An operation is clearly necessary when it is the only way to cure a life-threatening disease or condition. An operation is also indicated whenever the quality of life can be improved only by such measures. When misery or pain becomes unbearable, it would not be humane to persist with nonsurgical treatments if a surgical option existed. These general reasons for surgery are widely accepted.

But what about a host of other conditions that do not directly threaten a person's life or immediate well-being. Are hernia repairs unnecessary if the hernia causes no symptoms? Since only a small number of patients with unrepaired hernias will develop bowel obstruction and intestinal gangrene, is surgery designed to prevent those complications "unnecessary"? What about cosmetic surgery to remove a disfiguring birthmark? Is it "unnecessary" for such individuals to have plastic surgery to improve their appearance and sense of well-being, which could increase their chances of finding and keeping a job?

The decision to recommend surgery should be within the province of the surgeon. But the right to refuse surgery always remains with the patient. Pressures from patients or from referring physicians to perform inappropriate operations should be and are rejected by ethical surgeons. By virtue of extensive training and experience, only the surgeon is best qualified to judge whether surgery is truly indicated in an individual case and which type of operation should be done.

How can you protect yourself from the possibility of "unnecessary surgery"? You have already learned how to find the good surgeons, and by applying those same principles you can avoid the incompetents and the opportunists.

But what about the occasional unethical surgeon, the "bad apple"? Is the public at the mercy of such rogues? The surgical community relies on a number of mechanisms for removing unprincipled, dishonest, or unethical surgeons from the practice of surgery. (These procedures are described in Chapter 13.)

SECOND OPINIONS: ARE THEY WORTH IT?

If, after you meet with your proposed surgeon and discuss your options, you remain uncertain as to whether surgery is really necessary, or you're still unconvinced that the recommended operation is best for you, there's another alternative. If you decide you want another opinion, you should tell the first surgeon that you still have doubts about the necessity for surgery or the choice of operations, and you wish to get another surgeon's opinion. This does not in any way reflect on the integrity of the first surgeon but merely states that you have some doubts that you need to have resolved. You should not be embarrassed about this, nor should the surgeon take any offense at your suggestion. If you feel any resistance on the part of the surgeon to this suggestion, you should definitely find another surgeon.

A competent surgeon should never be threatened by another surgeon's opinion. In fact, a surgeon may want a second opinion if he or she has doubts about a proposed course of treatment. In essence, second opinions are only a form of consultation. Doctors do "sidewalk consults" all the time—in elevators, on the wards, in cafeterias, everywhere. The willingness of physicians to consult fellow surgeons is characteristic of professionals who put the welfare of the patient above their own ego.

Recently, however, because of the hue and cry over rising medical costs and concerns about unnecessary surgery, a number of large insurance companies have made second surgical opinions mandatory. Patients who participate in these plans must obtain a second opinion whenever certain surgical procedures are suggested. By requiring two independent surgeons to agree on a proposed operation, insurers hoped to reduce the incidence of unnecessary surgery. Should the patient fail to obtain a second surgical opinion, the insurance carrier will either refuse to reimburse the patient's expenses or will drastically reduce payments for the procedure.

Do mandatory second surgical opinions result in fewer operations? At this writing, it does not appear that they do. Continuing research on the number of operations performed, the costs and fees incurred, and the quality of care delivered will be necessary before that question can be answered. However, many conventional insurance plans no longer require mandatory second surgical opinions. According to the Health Insurance Association of America, the number of individual subscribers required to submit to a mandatory second surgical opinion fell from 53 percent in 1989 to 40 percent in 1992. During that time, many insurance companies discovered that it cost them more to obtain a verifying second surgical opinion than the company saved by avoiding unnecessary surgery. This observation is even more remarkable when you realize that charges for second opinions are approximately one tenth the fee for the proposed operation.

Although going for a second surgical opinion may be inconvenient and time-consuming, you should regard it as an opportunity to strengthen your own resolve. If the second opinion mirrors the first, you'll feel more certain of the need for surgery. It would certainly make sense for you to obtain a second opinion if you have any reason to doubt the qualifications of a proposed surgeon.

WHAT TO DO WHEN OPINIONS CONFLICT

What do you do if the surgeon giving the second opinion disagrees with the first, and either feels that surgery is not indicated at all or recommends another operation?

Doctors do disagree. Usually, disagreements between surgeons over the proper course of treatment arise from honest differences of opinion. Disagreements over whether surgery is necessary, or whether one particular operation is superior to another, are often the result of how each surgeon sees the case. When two surgeons disagree, you should not automatically assume that one of them is suggesting unnecessary surgery. As noted, indications for surgery are often not clearly defined; they may require considerable surgical judgment, and surgeons may differ widely in those judgments. What should you do if you're faced with differing surgical opinions?

First of all, if both surgeons are highly qualified, ask for detailed reasons as to why they have come to their particular opinions. You should also request that the consultants discuss your case with each other. Often, this is enough to resolve any differences in opinion, and also serves to limit repetition of lab tests, records, and X-ray examinations. If for any reason there is still disagreement, you can seek a third consultation with a well-recognized surgical expert. Your doctor should be able to suggest one or two in your area.

You will have to make the final decision. Get all the information you can, ask questions about everything you don't understand, and take your time (if you have that option). If something doesn't seem right to you, it may not be right. Don't proceed with surgery if you have doubts. An operation that is suggested "out of the blue," one for which you have had little preparation, should be carefully considered. Surgery for something that you consider trivial, an extensive and complicated operation, or a new and unproved procedure are all examples of situations requiring close examination. Use your common sense. Ask your primary care physician for advice. Even though you may not know everything about surgery, no one knows more about you than you do.

HOW TO CHANGE SURGEONS

Suppose you become dissatisfied with the surgeon chosen either by you or by your doctor. For whatever reasons, this individual has not lived up to your expectations. It is never in your best interest to keep quiet and go along with someone you do not like or trust.

It's probably wise to consider changing surgeons when there is a personality conflict or, for some reason, you have lost confidence in the surgeon. Although serious personality conflicts may occur between surgeons and patients, few patients wish to risk angering their surgeon. On occasion, a surgeon may decide not to treat a patient because of a personality conflict. Such a patient should then be referred to another surgeon. If direct discussion doesn't help, consult your doctor about how to find a satisfactory match.

If you prefer, you can ask your present surgeon to arrange for another surgeon to consider your case. The current surgeon is honor-bound and legally responsible for helping you find a suitable replacement. Furthermore, your care should be continued until the replacement is available. Failure to do this would constitute "abandonment," a situation for which the surgeon would be both ethically and legally accountable.

Suppose you don't want to switch to another surgeon, but you still have questions about the surgeon's plans for you or you continue to be dissatisfied with the care you have received. You have another option. You may request a consultation with another surgical specialist. (Check with your insurance company to see if this consultation would be covered.) This is not a second opinion, which is done prior to deciding on surgery and selecting a surgeon. The specialist will either dismiss your fears or confirm them. If the former, you can relax and proceed with the plan. If your concerns are confirmed by the consultant, you'll need to make a change. You should not hesitate to ask for a consultation or a change. After all, it's your body and your peace of mind.

UNNECESSARY SURGERY: DOES IT EXIST?

Is unnecessary surgery a fact? If surgeons know beforehand that an operation is unnecessary, there can be only one reason to go ahead and perform it anyway: money. Although the surgical profession is not riddled with avaricious opportunists who are beyond control, there are some in the medical profession who reject the idea that any unnecessary surgery exists.

"Unnecessary surgery" is surgery performed without any expectation of improving either the quality of a patient's life or the length of that life. Even with the best intentions, it may turn out that a given operation fails to produce the expected results. While, in one sense, this operation has proved to be "unnecessary," it is only unnecessary in hindsight.

Surgical decisions are made before the fact. And since surgery is not an exact science, such judgments will occasionally turn out to have been in error. As it is usually used, however, the phrase "unnecessary surgery" implies that surgeons know that certain operative procedures are not necessary but perform them anyway, thus subjecting patients to unnecessary risk and expense. There are dishonest and unethical people in all businesses and professions. Surgery is no exception. Such surgeons are a decided rarity, but they do exist.

Two operations frequently cited as examples of unnecessary surgery are tonsillectomy (removal of the tonsils) and hysterectomy (removal of the uterus). Today, there is little question that these operations have been overperformed in the past.

We now know that not all children need to have their tonsils removed. With advances in medical knowledge, more and more surgeons became aware that "routine" tonsillectomy was unnecessary, and the operation decreased in frequency. Similarly, the necessity for hysterectomy has declined with the use of alternative therapies.

As medical and surgical knowledge grows, there can be little doubt that some of the operations that we consider necessary today may well be unnecessary tomorrow. New developments may change existing recommendations. In fact, carotid artery surgery (to prevent strokes) and coronary bypass surgery (to prevent heart attacks) have recently been questioned. Several retrospective studies have suggested that as many as one third to one half of the patients undergoing carotid or coronary surgery can be treated equally well through nonsurgical means. The final answers are not yet in, but it appears that both coronary and carotid surgery will continue to be necessary in certain cases.

From a historical perspective, growth in our basic knowledge and development of new treatment alternatives regularly result in an overall reduction in the necessity for surgery. Once thorough evaluation has resulted in a recommendation for a change in treatment, such procedures are either restricted or discarded altogether. As better methods of therapy are conceived and become available, many outmoded operations are rejected by the surgical community.

Although not everyone will need to have their tonsils out, uterus removed, or blood vessels repaired, some people will need these operations for certain specific reasons. This is where surgical judgment comes in. Surgeons are well aware that the indications for certain operations change with new information, and those who remain current with the new information in their specialty are more aware of this than others. You can easily appreciate how important it is for your surgeon to remain up to date. It is estimated that the surgical information base completely turns over every six years. As a result, if your proposed surgeon does not participate in continuing medical education programs—by attending professional meetings or reading surgical journals or making rounds at a teaching hospital—you may be placing yourself in the hands of someone whose knowledge and skills have become obsolete.

8

SURGICAL FEES

Affordable health care is becoming an increasing concern for every American. Although surgical fees are a relative bargain compared to other health-care costs, having risen only half as much as the consumer price index from 1980 to 1992, that's small consolation to those faced with the prospect of paying for complicated surgical procedures. Is there anything you can do to protect yourself?

NEGOTIATING FEES

In recent years, responsibility for payment of surgical fees has shifted away from individual patients to third-party payers such as insurance companies or federal and state governments. This has caused many individuals to pay little attention to the cost of their surgical care. But increasingly, health-insurance contracts now require copayments, deductibles, and exclusions, so people are now more attentive to surgical fees as their direct out-of-pocket expenses have risen. Moreover, surgical fees can directly affect how much you pay in insurance premiums or for membership in an HMO or managed-care plan. So it's important for you to ask about surgical fees before you have an operation or sign an insurance contract.

Few people have ever thought about negotiating fees with a surgeon. Most people rather naively think that such fees are more or less the same, regardless of the surgeon they choose to perform the operation. Not true! Surgical fees can vary among surgeons, even in the same community, by 100 percent or more for the same operation.

Does the higher fee mean a better surgeon and a better operation? Since most surgeons set their own fees in a relatively free market, there's no necessary relationship between surgical fees and the quality of surgical care provided. But competition for patients among surgeons is increasing. In effect, if you have a surgical condition, you're in a buyer's market. Surgeons practicing the same specialty are potential competitors, vying, however politely, with one another for patients. If the supply of surgical services exceeds patient demand, prices (fees) must decline.

If you're not covered by any form of insurance that reimburses you for surgical fees, you may be able to save yourself a considerable amount of money by negotiating your surgical fee prior to the proposed operation. In a 1988 study of surgeons in the New York/New Jersey area, almost four out of five surgeons were willing to reduce their fees when asked to do so. Savings ranged from 25 to 35 percent, with the largest reductions being in the highest-priced procedures, such as coronary bypass and back surgery.

Even patients with insurance that provides surgical coverage can benefit from fee bargaining. Many policies include co-insurance, which amounts to 20 to 40 percent of the eligible surgical fee after you have satisfied the deductible; or a copayment, which makes you personally responsible for a fixed amount that you pay when you use a particular service. Then there is the balance, any amount in excess of the "usual and customary" fee allowed by the insurer. By negotiating with your surgeon up front, you may be able to reduce some or all of those out-of-pocket costs.

Should you try fee bargaining? If you have an uncomplicated surgical condition, fee bargaining with a competent surgeon makes good economic sense. Your condition is straightforward and can be handled by any number of competent surgeons, some of whom may be willing to negotiate their fees. However, if you have a complex condition, or if your situation is otherwise complicated, you need an expert surgeon. Here the laws of supply and demand work against you. There are rarely enough expert surgeons to go around.

You may be fortunate enough to have a surgeon who makes it a practice to reduce or even eliminate fees in situations of financial hardship. But unless you specifically ask for such consideration, you won't know, since surgeons rarely volunteer this information. Many surgeons are willing to set up a payment schedule tailored to your needs, including monthly payment options. Most surgeons are reasonable: You can talk to them about money. Frank discussions are appropriate—and expected.

To give you some guidelines with which to negotiate fees, Table 8.1 lists median and high fees for the 48 surgical procedures performed most frequently in 1993.

TABLE 8.1

Median and High Surgical Fees, National Averages (1993)

Fee research from Medirisk, Inc., of Atlanta, Georgia, derived from and validated by the company's proprietary database containing more than 450 million current claims transaction records.

	MEDIAN	HIGH
Obstetrical Procedures		
Episiotomy	$ 255	$ 510
Cesarean section	2,201	5,522
Gastrointestinal Procedures		
Gastrointestinal endoscopy		
Esophagogastroduodenoscopy	607	1,096
ERCP	889	1,632
Colonoscopy	823	1,341
Cholecystectomy		
Conventional	1,964	4,074
Laparoscopic	2,317	3,890
Lysis of adhesions	1,872	3,355
Appendectomy		
Conventional	1,186	2,729
Laparoscopic	1,386	2,318
Colectomy	2,569	4,777

TABLE 8.1 (cont'd.)

Median and High Surgical Fees, National Averages (1993)

	MEDIAN	HIGH
Inguinal herniorrhaphy		
Conventional	1,215	2,711
Laparoscopic	1,460*	3,250*
Cardiovascular Procedures		
Cardiac catheterization	$500	$1,149
Coronary artery bypass graft (2)	6,640	9,273
Pacemaker implantation	1,958	3,213
Blood vessel surgery		
Aneurysmectomy	4,384	7,263
Aortofemoral bypass	4,250	7,323
Femoropopliteal bypass	3,150	6,000
Arteriovenous fistula	664	1,018
Musculoskeletal Procedures		
Arthroscopy (knee)	969	1,954
Open reduction—internal fixation		
Humerus	1,846	4,646
Femur	2,607	4,439
Arthroplasty		
Hip (total)	4,796	8,224
Knee	3,775	5,231
Spinal fusion (lumbar)	4,179	8,463
Intervertebral diskectomy	3,647	8,031
Gynecological Surgery		
Dilation and curettage	680	1,317
Hysterectomy		
Abdominal	2,355	6,453
Vaginal	2,330	5,678

*Data from author's independent survey

TABLE 8.1 (cont'd.)

Median and High Surgical Fees, National Averages (1993)

	MEDIAN	HIGH
Salpingo-oophorectomy	1,559	3,365
Tubal ligation/destruction		
Conventional	$1,233	$2,707
Laparoscopic	1,245	2,295
Repair of pelvic hernia	2,093	4,104
Genitourinary Procedures		
Cystoscopy	511	923
Prostatectomy		
TURP	2,512	4,864
Retropubic	2,623	5,707
Radical perineal	3,019	6,065
Skin Surgery		
Skin biopsy	70	152
Skin graft (free flap)	6,716	13,172
Breast Surgery		
Lumpectomy	657	1,720
Simple mastectomy	1,293	2,370
Modified radical mastectomy	2,055	4,373
Thoracic Surgery		
Bronchoscopy and biopsy	574	1,247
Lung resection		
Lobectomy	2,835	5,555
Pneumonectomy	3,489	6,587
Central Nervous System Surgery		
Craniotomy for tumor	5,821	10,872
Eye Surgery		
Cataract extraction with insertion of intraocular lens	2,594	3,890

ASSIGNMENT

If Medicare is your primary insurance and you wish to limit surgical fees, the concept of assignment is critical for you to understand. As an independent contractor to the federal government for the care of Medicare patients, any surgeon who chooses to treat Medicare patients has the option to accept or reject "assignment." Accepting assignment means agreeing to accept as full payment whatever amount Part B of Medicare calculates, or "assigns," for a particular procedure. Medicare will then pay 80 percent of that charge, and the patient is responsible for the remaining 20 percent. It is actually illegal for the surgeon not to bill for the additional 20 percent.

If the surgeon "rejects assignment," the patient can be billed for any portion of the surgical fee in excess of the Medicare allowance (up to a certain maximum amount) for that particular surgical procedure. Such extra billing, when the surgeon rejects assignment, is called "balance billing." Clearly, it's in your financial interest to find a surgeon who is willing to accept assignment. Failure to discover whether or not your surgeon accepts assignment could leave you open to balance billing. If you're in doubt as to whether your surgeon accepts assignment, ask. Physicians and surgeons who always accept assignment are also listed in the *Medicare Participating Physicians Directory,* available at your local Social Security office.

HMOs, PPOs, IPAs

A newer approach toward controlling physicians' fees and overall health-care costs has been the development of prepaid health plans. Under certain plans, physicians are paid a specific amount per patient per year (called "capitation"), regardless of whether the patient remains well or suffers catastrophic (expensive) illness. All medical expenses, including surgical fees, are taken from the initial payment. So it's in the financial interest of the physicians to emphasize preventive medicine and encourage members of those plans to stay well. Those plans are therefore called Health Maintenance Organizations (HMOs).

Other varieties of prepaid health plans include Preferred Provider Organizations (PPOs) and Independent Practice Associations (IPAs). In these plans, physicians offer discounted fees for service in return for large numbers of patients. In a PPO arrangement, hospitals and physicians individually contract with an employer, an insurance company, or a third-party payer to provide discounted services to subscribing patients. Patients are encouraged by the sponsoring organization to restrict their choice of physicians to those who agree to discount their fees (the preferred provider list, or "panel"). These doctors are not listed as "preferred" because they are necessarily outstanding, but because they have agreed to lower fees. Patients who choose to consult physicians not on the preferred list are usually held personally responsible for deductibles and co-insurance payments.

Variations of PPOs, such as managed-care systems, seek to control costs by negotiating fee schedules, conducting utilization and quality reviews, and including risk management, ambulatory care, nursing-home care, and other aspects of overall health care. Currently (1994), the federal Health Care Financing Administration (HCFA) is considering an alternative that would expand Medicare's participating physician program by creating regional federal PPOs.

Independent Practice Associations (IPAs) offer a different approach. In an IPA, a number of physicians join together to offer their services directly to employers, unions, social organizations, or any large patient group. Physicians negotiate fee schedules directly with the patient organization.

PPOs and IPAs are particularly attractive to employers, who have watched the costs of providing health-care benefits to their employees increase every year. Employer-sponsored health insurance plans now account for 60 percent of all privately purchased health care in the United States, an estimated $263 billion in 1993. Costs for providing medical benefits to employees continue to rise faster than inflation, and during 1991 amounted to an average of $4,255 per worker. As a result, more and more companies are requiring workers to help pay for their health care; 55 percent of 2,400 companies surveyed require workers to share costs. Hospitals, physicians, or joint ventures currently sponsor almost half of all existing PPOs, whereas insurance companies and Blue Cross/Blue Shield account for another third.

Do these prepaid health plans work? Are they saving companies money when compared with more traditional, private, fee-for-service plans, such as Blue Cross/Blue Shield? Recent studies have failed to validate claims that managed health care systems have actually resulted in overall cost savings to society, or that they have improved the quality of care. However, since these systems have been in operation for only a relatively short time, it's perhaps more fair to say that the jury is still out.

What does all of this mean to you, the consumer? If you choose to enroll in a prepaid health plan as a private subscriber, be aware that your choice of doctors is limited to those physicians who have joined the plan. If for any reason you need a surgeon who is not a member of the plan, you may have to pay a part or, in some plans, all of the surgical fee out of your own pocket. This restriction in choosing your own physician becomes even more burdensome when your condition requires a highly specialized surgeon (see Chapter 6).

Limitation in your choice of physicians and surgeons is the principal disadvantage of managed-care systems and constitutes the sacrifice you may have to make to reduce your monthly health-care expenses. But managed health care plans can result in considerable savings in copayments and deductibles for care actually received. With such plans, copayments are low and deductibles are often absent. The reverse is true with traditional health insurance.

Another disadvantage with some managed-care plans is a potential limit on patients' access to medical and surgical care. In some plans, patients have to wait longer for appointments than they would for care under traditional insurance plans. In some cases, this is because so few doctors are available in a particular plan; in others—particularly plans in which primary-care physicians get a "capitation" payment designed to cover all the health-care needs of the patients assigned to them—delays may be attributable to the financial incentive such physicians may feel to undertreat or limit the services provided.

But one cannot generalize about prepaid health plans. Marked differences abound regarding monthly charges, payments and deductibles, the quality of participating doctors and hospitals, and the management of the plans. Patient satisfaction with prepaid health care plans varies widely and is dependent upon the individual plan. When choosing a plan, therefore, it's vitally important for you to compare not only costs but coverage and the quality of physicians and surgeons included in the plan. In August 1992, *Consumer Reports* listed some important questions to ask about any plan you're thinking of signing up with:

1. When must I notify the plan before going to the hospital or when an emergency occurs, and how do I do it? Some managed-care plans require you to obtain approval before going to a hospital; in others, such as HMOs and PPOs, your doctor usually obtains permission for you. If you ignore the rules, you could jeopardize your benefits.
2. Will I be penalized for going outside the network? Your share of the costs can vary, depending on the kind of plan you choose. But just knowing the cost-sharing amounts isn't enough. You need to know how they are applied. If your plan covers 90 percent of the cost, does that 90 percent apply to the doctor's actual charge or to what the plan determines is an allowable charge? If the doctor charges $8,000 but the plan allows only $3,000 for a procedure, you would receive only $2,400 (80 percent of $3,000) and still owe the doctor $5,600.
3. What happens if I see a specialist who is not in the plan? That may happen if you belong to a PPO. If your primary-care doctor refers you to an in-plan specialist, you usually get the high "in-network" benefits. If you choose an out-of-plan specialist, you may get lower benefits.
4. Are all services offered by a doctor in a network covered? A plan may authorize a doctor to perform routine gynecology but not infertility treatment, for example.
5. Who pays if my regular doctor is unavailable and another doctor is covering? Will the covering physician be

able to collect from the managed-care plan, or will he or she bill me for payment?

6. Are doctors in the plan taking any new patients? Look skeptically at plans whose directories indicate that many of the listed doctors are not taking additional patients. The HMO or PPO organization may be keeping those doctors in its directory simply to make the book look fatter, or the doctors may be dissatisfied with the plan and not want to accept any new patients from among its members.

7. Are the doctors who belong to the plan board certified (meaning that they've passed certain tests for competency in their medical field)? Have they been with the plan long? Are there grievances or complaints against them? The HMO or PPO may be reluctant to tell you, so be persistent.

8. Is the doctor I'm considering satisfied with the plan? Call and ask. If doctors are unhappy, either because they are not paid in a timely fashion or for other reasons, you probably don't want to pick that doctor. A dissatisfied doctor may be on the verge of dropping out, which would disrupt your care.

9. What is the doctor's obligation to me if he or she leaves the plan while I'm in the hospital? The plan may require the doctor to continue your treatment until you're discharged.

10. If my employer asks me to switch plans during the course of treatment or during a pregnancy, can I stay with my current physician until the treatment or the pregnancy is completed? Some plans will allow you to do that, others won't.

11. How does the plan handle mental-health coverage? What are the benefits?

12. Who determines the care I will receive—the organization itself or a utilization-review company it hires?
13. What recourse do I have if I'm unhappy with my care?

The time and effort you spend in evaluating and choosing a plan may produce big dividends if you ever need expensive surgical care.

9

CHOOSING A HOSPITAL

The hospital you go to for your operation can materially affect the outcome of your surgery. Many people realize that hospitals differ from one another, but most are not aware of why these differences exist or how important they may be. Among the most significant reasons why certain hospitals are better for you than others is the simple fact that not all hospitals are staffed or equipped to perform all operations equally well.

With the recent changes in health-care financing, more and more hospitals are becoming increasingly specialized in an effort to hold down costs. Medical and surgical equipment has become enormously expensive, and the ability to provide the necessary equipment for all surgical procedures is becoming limited to only large and very well financed institutions. Furthermore, labor costs continue to rise. Having enough specialized technicians, assistants, and nurses to aid and ensure your recovery has become a luxury in many hospitals.

Referral hospitals (those to which patients requiring specialized procedures are sent) attract surgeons expert in those special areas. They are at the forefront of developments in their own, often narrow, areas of interest and can apply the most up-to-date approach to your condition. Surgery, and any other skill requiring highly developed eye-hand coordination, gets easier and is better performed when it is practiced frequently. The staff of a referral hospital, by its very nature, gets concentrated experience in the management of special cases.

What if you have some underlying condition, such as heart disease or diabetes, that makes your proposed surgical procedure more risky than it would be for a healthy individual? If that's the case, you will need the kind of continuous highly specialized care usually found in larger, more sophisticated hospitals. Such care is given in intensive care units (ICUs) by highly trained personnel using state-of-the-art monitoring equipment. In brief, having the right hospital can be almost as important as having the right surgeon. Don't let considerations of distance stand in your way. It is far better to have a long trip to an inconveniently located hospital than to risk the possibility of mistakes being made in a nearby but less qualified institution.

SUPPORT PERSONNEL

The importance of a hospital's auxiliary health-care personnel cannot be overemphasized. Your surgeon may see you twice a day during the time you are in the hospital. If each visit lasts 15 minutes, who takes care of you the other 23½ hours each day? What if you experience an emergency complication after your operation? Your surgeon may be busy with another patient or not even in the hospital. In such a case, a full-time staff physician or a member of the resident house staff on call in the hospital 24 hours a day could make the difference between life and death for you.

One of the most dangerous things to happen to you during your hospital stay is being anesthetized before surgery. All sleep-producing drugs and pain-killing agents interrupt bodily functions. Improperly given, general anesthesia can result in death. Fortunately, there are physicians who have chosen to specialize in this field, thereby reducing the risk. Unfortunately, however, there are not enough anesthesiologists to go around. Other, less well trained personnel—nurses, physicians' assistants, and general physicians—also administer anesthesia and are known as anesthetists. Notice the difference between anesthesiologists and anesthetists: anesthesiologists are specialized doctors, anesthetists are not. In the better hospitals, staff anesthesiologists administer anesthesia themselves or supervise lesser-trained anesthetists. Such supervision should rarely extend beyond two or three simultaneous operations. If those conditions do not exist where you plan to have your surgery, be aware that you are at increased risk. That's not to suggest in any way that many nurse anesthetists and physicians' assistants cannot manage complicated cases, or do not give exemplary anesthesia, but rather to point out the importance of determining who will put you to sleep and monitor your vital signs during and immediately after your operation.

We have already touched on the importance of specialized personnel when your condition is (or becomes) complicated. Having the right person available immediately is often lifesaving. The more serious your condition, or the more complicated your proposed surgery, the more you need highly skilled backup personnel on a 24-hour basis. Life-support teams for cardiac arrest have a two-minute maximum response time in hospitals geared to the management of difficult surgical cases. Since irreversible brain damage begins to develop as quickly as four minutes after blood flow stops, you can appreciate the importance of immediate availability. Equally important are the training and experience of the various physicians whom your surgeon might need to call in for consultation on postoperative problems.

THREE CLASSES OF HOSPITALS

Ideally, we would all like to have our operation done by the best surgeon working in the best hospital. Besides being impractical, such wishes are probably not medically necessary in most cases. Many surgical procedures are neither complex nor demanding of highly specialized surgical expertise or state-of-the-art hospital facilities.

Most prospective patients are not aware that they can sometimes have a voice in the choice of a hospital. Many surgeons have admitting privileges in more than one hospital and can therefore accommodate your preferences—if you express them. On the other hand, your health-care insurance plan or HMO may severely limit your choice of institutions. If you do have a choice, the trick is to know when expert surgeons and sophisticated hospital facilities are needed. There are a number of criteria you can apply to make these determinations.

As a general rule, if the proposed operation can be performed under local anesthesia without hospitalization (ambulatory, same-day, outpatient, or "walk-in" surgery), the operation is not likely to require sophisticated hospital facilities. Those procedures can be performed in any hospital accredited by the Joint Commission for Accreditation of Healthcare Organizations (JCAHO). If your hospital is accredited, it will display a certificate from JCAHO. If you don't see it, ask for it.

This generalization often holds true even when small amounts of general anesthesia (less than one hour) are necessary. Examples of such procedures are cataract surgery, the drainage of abscesses, uterine dilation and curettage, most biopsies, setting simple fractures, abortions, small skin grafts, tubal ligation, vasectomy, and minor arm or leg surgery.

This same criterion may be applied to the selection of a surgeon. The level of surgical training is so good in this country that ordinary uncomplicated surgery, which can be performed under local anesthesia, does not often require highly qualified, specialized surgeons. Thus, as a general rule, the type of anesthesia to be used for the operation may dictate the level of surgical expertise as well as the hospital sophistication that will be required. To oversimplify, perhaps, one might say that if you're going to need local anesthesia, in most cases a local general surgeon and a local community hospital will be all you'll need.

TIER ONE PROCEDURES

Eye surgery (cataracts)
Ear surgery
Minor biopsies of surface organs
Minor arm and leg surgery

Hernia surgery (groin)
Drainage of infections
Dilation and curettage (D & C)
Tubal ligation
Termination of pregnancy
Vasectomy
Small skin grafts

A second tier of operations can be grouped around the need for general or spinal anesthesia. These are cases that are either more extensive or require more time to perform. Surgical procedures requiring general anesthesia may or may not require specialized services. Most local accredited hospitals and competent board certified surgeons are equipped to perform routine, uncomplicated neck, abdominal, hernia, blood-vessel, back, and gynecologic surgery.

TIER TWO PROCEDURES

Neck surgery (thyroid, parathyroid)
Breast surgery
Abdominal surgery
Herniorrhaphy (abdominal)
Blood vessel surgery
Amputations
Cosmetic surgery
Prostate surgery
Hysterectomy
Vaginal surgery
Bone and joint surgery
Disk surgery

The key word here is *uncomplicated*. Uncomplicated surgical conditions make up the overwhelming number of reasons for surgery in this country. Because this is true, your local hospital and a competent surgeon are quite capable of delivering quality care for Tier Two cases.

But even common surgical conditions can become complicated. In the presence of complications, a higher level of surgical expertise and care is required and a more sophisticated hospital should be sought. If you're in doubt about whether your condition is complicated, ask your internist or primary-care physician, or the surgeon to whom you have been referred.

HOW CAN YOU TELL IF A HOSPITAL IS EQUIPPED TO MEET YOUR NEEDS?

There are several yardsticks that you can use. First, if your condition is rare; if you have developed complications; if the surgical procedure is difficult; if you have significant heart, lung, kidney, or liver disease in addition to the reason for the surgery, then you will probably be better off in a sophisticated referral hospital. In general, larger hospitals, with more than 500 beds, can support a full range of health-care specialists, including expert surgeons, and are accustomed to handling complicated or otherwise difficult cases. While this is another oversimplification, and exceptions do occur in both directions, the size of a hospital is often a measure of its ability to handle more complicated cases. But note that there are many community hospitals with state-of-the-art facilities and a highly trained professional staff capable of dealing with a wide range of medical or surgical problems.

Second, most hospitals affiliated with a university or a medical school—teaching hospitals—are capable of dealing with the widest range of surgical needs, from sewing a laceration to heart transplantation. In a teaching hospital, medical interns, residents, and research fellows handle much of the medical care—under the close supervision of an attending physician or professor who is usually board certified in one or more specialties. University-affiliated hospitals are often referral centers to which community physicians and surgeons send their more specialized cases. Since universities have research and teaching functions, hospitals affiliated with them are often at the forefront of medical knowledge and practice. In fact, one recent study, using data adjusted for severity of illness, found that the overall death rate for patients was lowest in hospitals affiliated with university medical schools and in which residents assisted university attendings in patient care.

This should not be interpreted to mean that everyone needs to be cared for at a university hospital. Your local hospital is quite capable of handling uncomplicated Tier One and Tier Two surgical procedures. In fact, many university hospitals don't do as good a job with uncomplicated minor surgery as a local hospital might do. Their emphasis on the complicated and the difficult may cause them to pay less attention to the needs of a patient with a routine appendectomy, for example.

While the great majority of surgical cases fall into the first or second tier of difficulty, there is a small but significant group of procedures for which highly trained and specialized surgeons and sophisticated hospital facilities are required (Tier Three procedures).

TIER THREE PROCEDURES

Brain and spinal-cord surgery
Head and neck cancer surgery
Heart surgery

Lung surgery
Liver surgery
Pancreas surgery
Microsurgery
Organ transplantation
Severe burns
Severe trauma
Surgery in the newborn
Reoperations in severely ill patients
Complicated, complex, or rare conditions

Common sense tells us that these complicated surgical procedures should be carried out only in those referral hospitals that routinely deal with such cases, where the staff and the facilities are equal to the demands of the task at hand.

EVALUATING A HOSPITAL

At first, the task of evaluating a hospital may seem daunting, but there are criteria by which any hospital can be judged. Here are some basic questions you can ask when you're trying to see if your proposed hospital measures up.

1. Is It Accredited?

Accreditation by the JCAHO cannot guarantee that a hospital is first rate, but it can help safeguard against substandard medical care and a hazardous physical plant. There is no legal requirement that a hospital or any other type of health-care facility be accredited. But the fact that a facility is accredited by the JCAHO indicates that it has voluntarily met established strict standards for its operation and for the delivery of care and services.

If a hospital wants to be accredited, it must conform to a set of published standards in every aspect of its operation. The first step is for the hospital to submit an application. After a detailed questionnaire has been completed, the hospital receives an on-site survey by a team composed of a physician and either a hospital administrator or a registered nurse (or all three).

The JCAHO team makes an extensive examination of the hospital. They ascertain whether the physical plant is properly maintained to meet safety requirements. They verify ownership of the hospital to determine who is ultimately responsible for the facility's performance. They check the bylaws and decide whether the medical staff follows them. They seek to determine whether the medical staff is functioning effectively and whether its performance is of the quality necessary to deliver good care.

Particular emphasis is placed on the adequacy and comprehensiveness of the medical records, and on a review of medical staff organization. The team meets with members of the hospital staff and examines patient records and the minutes of staff and committee meetings. They inquire into the way privileges are granted and delineated.

The hospital's provisions for monitoring its own performance and its procedures for self-evaluation are also studied by the survey team. The quality of medical care can be judged from the completeness of patients' medical charts, the frequency with which mortality review committees meet, and the details covered in those meetings. The survey team examines the records of peer-review committees, organized to determine inconsistencies and deficiencies in the management of patients and to guard against the abuse of hospital privileges, as well as the records of staff utilization committees, which determine whether available bed space is being used efficiently.

In checking each service and department, the survey team evaluates the hospital's documented evidence that it is conforming to JCAHO standards. The evaluation includes not only the medical records department but also the laboratories; the X-ray, nursing, and dietary services; the departments of anesthesiology and, if the hospital has them, the departments of physical medicine, pharmacy, medical social services, and emergency services.

When the on-site survey is completed, the team submits its report and recommendations to the JCAHO Hospital Accreditation Program. After an overall review, the hospital may receive one of three ratings: two-year accreditation, one-year accreditation, or no accreditation. The decision is then communicated to the hospital, together with recommendations for improvement. Hospitals given accreditation usually display their certificate in the lobby. But if you're uncertain whether a hospital is accredited, you can find out by asking the hospital administrators or by writing to JCAHO, 875 North Michigan Avenue, Chicago, IL 60611.

Since accreditation is voluntary, the fact that a hospital is not accredited may simply mean that it has not sought accreditation. But unless you have good reason to do otherwise, you should avoid, if possible, any nonaccredited hospital.

2. Is It a Teaching Hospital?

We have already touched on the advantages of a teaching hospital. What that means is that it has a formal program for the training of medical personnel. The higher the level of such teaching, the higher the level of medical services the hospital is likely to provide. The best indicator of a good teaching program is affiliation with a medical school. Hospitals with such affiliation are likely to have available as needed the services of qualified generalists and specialists in all fields; they often have full-time staff physicians in charge of key departments; and they attract many of the best young physicians who want residency training in the specialties. Such an environment is also likely to bring out the best in the doctors and other personnel affiliated with the hospital.

3. Who Owns the Hospital?

The third major question to ask about a hospital concerns its ownership: Is it a voluntary, nonprofit, or community hospital? Is it a privately owned, proprietary hospital? Or is it a third type, sponsored by the municipal, county, state, or federal government?

Although the voluntary and proprietary hospitals generally tend to follow different patterns, the relationship between the quality of medical care in a hospital and its type of ownership is less direct than is the case with accreditation or teaching services. But in the judgment of many experts, the voluntary hospital, when one has a choice, is to be preferred.

On the whole, government-supported hospitals also offer good medical facilities and competent staff. In those instances in which government-sponsored hospitals are affiliated with top-rated medical schools, the facilities and the staff may be superb. However, these institutions may fall behind voluntary hospitals in such matters as luxury accommodations and the number of private rooms.

The voluntary hospital is a nonprofit community institution functioning under religious or other voluntary auspices. The organizational structure of a voluntary nonprofit hospital, ideally, is designed to protect the patient in every possible way. Ultimate responsibility for all that takes place in such a hospital rests with its board of trustees, generally selected from among the community's business and professional people, who serve without pay. To manage the hospital, the trustees appoint a paid administrator, increasingly in recent years someone specially trained in the field of hospital administration, rather than a physician.

The proprietary hospitals are, in effect, commercial establishments, offering a special service to the public. The basic objectives of such institutions are less clear-cut and less open to generalization. They are, of course, intended to help sick people. But they are also profit-making institutions, and the degree of their dedication to profit varies markedly. It must be said, of course, that even a high degree of dedication to profit does not preclude high-quality medical care, any more than the nonprofit motive of community or voluntary hospitals assures good care.

Like the voluntary and proprietary hospitals, those sponsored by state and local governments vary widely in quality. The category of tax-supported institutions includes some very large hospitals as well as some much smaller ones. All such institutions may sometimes be compelled to curtail services when budget allocations are cut. Publicly funded hospitals share a distinctive mission: They provide medical services for the indigent. Of course, any sick person, regardless of need, may be admitted to such hospitals, but the nonindigent patient is usually billed according to standard rates.

As far as internal workings are concerned, one important factor differentiates the three types of hospital. In the best of the voluntary hospitals, there are strict provisions for inspection, evaluation, and control of the medical activities of affiliated doctors. Government-sponsored institutions also tend to have rigid standards. On the whole, proprietary institutions are the least thorough concerning inspection, evaluation, and other standards. For example, in proprietary hospitals there are apt to be fewer restrictions on the scope of surgery performed by general practitioners. This means that in those hospitals it may be easier for physicians to perform operations they are not qualified to perform.

Attractive surroundings—a recently painted interior, modern fixtures, and the like—can be reassuring and desirable in a hospital, but the real worth of a hospital lies in the capabilities of its attending staff and the adequacy and competency of such basic ancillary services as the pathology department, the chemistry laboratory, and the radiology section. Your physician will make a diagnosis and formulate therapy on the basis of reports from those areas. The reliability of such reports is crucial in determining the real value of a hospital.

10

PAIN CONTROL

Pain is a mechanism for protection of the organism. When we experience pain, our attention is immediately drawn to where the pain is felt. All our efforts are concentrated on removing the affected part from the painful stimulus or otherwise achieving relief.

For many people, however, the mere thought of the pain likely to result from surgery produces anxiety and delay in acceptance. But for those who have been procrastinating because of the fear of surgical pain, there is good news: Recent advances in pain control and anesthesia have markedly reduced the amount of pain surgical patients must endure. If fear of pain has prevented you from having necessary surgery, it's now time for you to reconsider.

ANESTHESIA

As we noted in our brief discussion of the history of surgery, control of pain was one of the conditions necessary for surgery's full development. Anesthesia (the total absence of pain) was first performed in 1842 by a rural Georgia physician using diethyl ether as the anesthetic agent while removing an ovarian cyst. Soon after, a better-publicized event took place at Massachusetts General Hospital, where a dentist anesthetized a patient so that a surgeon could painlessly remove a tumor from the patient's jaw. Later, a second dentist permitted an itinerant showman to administer nitrous oxide gas to him while a third dentist painlessly removed one of his molars. With these and similar demonstrations, the era of anesthesia had begun.

General Anesthesia

Until recently, inhalational gases, such as ether and nitrous oxide, were the only effective anesthetic agents. Today, gases derived from vapors of liquid fluorinated carbons have become almost ideal inhalation agents. When compared to the inhalation agents in use just a generation ago, modern anesthetic agents, such as desfluorane, enflurane, and isoflurane, have minimal risk of accidentally exploding or damaging the patient in any way.

The object of all general anesthesia agents is total unconsciousness. That includes not only the total absence of pain but also complete relaxation of all muscles and complete amnesia for everything that happened while surgery was being performed. Sodium pentothal, injected into a vein, achieves those results very quickly and effectively; however, its effects last only about 15 minutes, so it is often used to "put you under" before the continuous administration of anesthetic gases begins. Exactly how the various inhalational anesthetic agents achieve pain control is not known, but we do know that anesthetic agents cause a reversible blockade of nerve-impulse transmission.

Recovery from inhalation-induced general anesthesia is the reverse of its induction. Since modern anesthetic agents are not metabolized in the body, your body gets rid of them the same way it received them—by breathing: You exhale the gases from your lungs. It takes some time for them to pass from the many body tissues, where the gases may have been stored, into the blood and from there to the lungs, where they are finally exhaled. That's why recovery from general anesthesia is often slow and why it's necessary to go to a recovery room, where you can be closely observed while the gas leaves your body and you return to full conscioueness.

It is rare today for anyone to attempt to achieve all the desired goals for general anesthesia by using a single inhalational agent. More often, individual anesthetic agents are combined with other drugs, such as barbiturates, to retard nerve transmission; benzodiazepines to produce amnesia of the events surrounding surgery; neuromuscular relaxants to diminish muscle tone; and opiates to dilute the concentration of anesthetic agents. As a result, the administration of general anesthesia has become increasingly complex. Balancing all those drugs together, each with its own limitations and dangers, while simultaneously maintaining a level of anesthesia sufficient for surgery and constantly monitoring organ function, has become both a difficult science and a real art.

You should also understand that all inhalational anesthetic agents and anesthetic drug adjuncts are depressives: To some degree, they all diminish the function of important organs. Too much depression of function can be fatal. So it's neither safe nor desirable for you to be asleep before you get to the operating room. A patient who arrives at the hospital and says "Knock me out and don't wake me up till it's all over" is asking for trouble. Fortunately, that kind of request won't be honored.

Of the 30 million general anesthetics administered annually in the United States, fewer than 0.01 percent result in death; that's 1 fatality in 10,000 procedures. While this may be a small number, it is real. Moreover, it has been estimated that of the 2,500 deaths directly attributable to anesthesia each year in this country, more than half are preventable.

In addition to the general depressive action of inhalational anesthetics on bodily functions, some notable short-term side effects may occur. Nausea and occasional retching may be seen in approximately 10 to 20 percent of patients awakening from general anesthesia. One of the main reasons why you will not be allowed to eat for some hours before surgery is that if you should vomit, some gastric contents might enter the windpipe while you're asleep. Aspiration, as that is called, can be very dangerous.

Longer-term side effects of inhalational agents are almost nonexistent. Although it was once thought that there was some danger of liver damage following administration of the anesthetic gas halothane, intensive investigations have failed to establish any conclusive link between modern inhalational agents and organ damage of any kind, provided the gases are administered correctly and within recommended dosages. In short, modern inhalational anesthesia is safe when properly given.

Regional Anesthesia

Unlike general anesthesia, regional anesthesia does not put you to sleep. Since it doesn't involve depression of the pain centers of the brain, you remain conscious. (In most cases, you'll be given some form of sedation as well, to help you relax and control anxiety.) Regional anesthesia confines its effects to a specific region of the body without affecting other areas, such as the heart, the lungs, or the brain. The anesthetic agent is injected directly to the nerves that serve the region of the body where the operation will be performed so that you will feel no pain until the anesthetic wears off. Some patients report feeling a sensation of painless pressure while the surgeon is working.

- For spinal anesthesia, the anesthetic is injected into the fluid surrounding the spinal cord. Sensation is thereby blocked for the region below the point at which the injection was given.
- For epidural anesthesia, the anesthetic is injected above the outer lining of the spinal cord. In contrast with a spinal block, epidural anesthesia can be reinjected through a catheter during a long procedure or even during the postoperative period.

Local Anesthesia

Local anesthesia, with agents such as tetracaine, lidocaine, and bupivacaine, is usually administered by needle injection into the immediate vicinity of the procedure. This is the method most people have experienced in the dentist's office.

Injection of regional and local anesthetics interrupts or suppresses the transmission of pain impulses by blocking the transfer of chemicals across the nerve membrane. Local anesthesia lasts from minutes to hours, and can be controlled by choosing the appropriate agent (short- or long-acting). Local anesthetics are broken down by enzymes in the body (metabolized) and excreted as inert breakdown products. That's why you experience a gradual return of sensation in the treated area as the anesthetic "wears off."

Given in appropriate quantities, local anesthetic agents are remarkably safe. However, if given to excess, they may produce some bad reactions. Convulsions occur in approximately 1 out of every 15,000 administrations of local anesthetic agents, and are easily treated when corrective therapy is prompt.

A common complication is "postspinal headache." It occurs in 20 to 30 percent of patients following regional spinal anesthesia. It's a minor self-limiting complication, usually lasting only a day or two, and is probably caused by a brief leak of spinal fluid. Headaches are less common with epidural anesthesia (1 to 5 percent).

An extremely rare complication of spinal anesthesia, total paralysis, occurs once in every 100,000 cases. Most of these episodes have been traced to defective agents or techniques. For all practical purposes, no significant risk for paralysis exists with modern agents and techniques for spinal anesthesia.

Choosing Your Anesthesia

In general, it's probably best if you leave the choice of the type of anesthesia up to your anesthesiologist. As a result of extensive training and practical experience, anesthesiologists are in the best position to weigh the merits of general versus regional anesthesia. Still, you should get a chance to discuss the options with your doctors, and the more you know about it, the better you'll be able to understand their decision.

Regional anesthesia is inherently safer than general anesthesia, and it is usually chosen for relatively minor operations, procedures on the extremities, or whenever it's important for the patient to be conscious. General anesthesia is chosen for more serious surgical procedures, operations upon the head, chest, or abdomen, or for prolonged and difficult operations (see Chapter 9). Local and regional anesthesia are preferred for most Tier One procedures and some Tier Two operations. General anesthesia is required for all Tier Three procedures.

Nevertheless, if you have strong negative feelings about spinal anesthesia, or its safer equivalents—epidural and caudal anesthesia—you should express them directly to the anesthesiologist. You will not be forced to have spinal anesthesia if you don't wish to.

Can you choose your anesthesiologist in the same way you choose your surgeon? Yes, but it's far more difficult. You can't rely on your primary-care physician for a recommendation, since anesthesiologists rarely interact with physicians other than surgeons. But surgeons do know who the "best" anesthesiologists are and can request that a specific individual be scheduled for your operation. Not all hospitals permit this; but if yours does, you might as well ask for the best.

ANALGESIA—POSTOPERATIVE PAIN CONTROL

As a patient having general anesthesia, the last thing you may remember clearly about the day of your surgery will be lying on the operating table before the anesthesiologist gave you the anesthetic agent. When you awaken, you'll be in the recovery room, but you'll remain drowsy from the residual effects of the anesthesia. It's here where you will first feel pain, as the anesthesia wears off and you begin to need analgesia. (To distinguish anesthesia from analgesia, you must know that analgesia is defined as "reduced sensibility to pain without loss of consciousness and without the sense of touch necessarily being affected.")

In the past, pain control after surgery was often inadequate, with many postoperative patients suffering excessively. The mainstay of postoperative pain control was intramuscular injection of a specified dose of narcotics, usually at intervals of three to four hours or (within limits) whenever the patient requested it. Considerable delay was often involved: The patient would call the nurse—often waiting until the pain was almost unbearable; the nurse would respond, then go to the locked narcotics cabinet, prepare the injection, and return to the patient's room to administer the dose. Since an intramuscular narcotic is absorbed in a cycle (initially delayed, rising to a peak, then declining over a two- to three-hour period), the narcotic is actually in the therapeutic range (its minimally effective analgesic concentration, or MEAC) for only a fraction of the four-hour interval between injections. As a result, patients receiving pain medication were on a roller-coaster of pain (a lot of pain, diminished pain, no pain, moderate pain, and a lot of pain) as the drug entered and left the bloodstream on its way to and from the pain-control centers in the brain.

Today, the concept of continuous postoperative pain control has been enthusiastically embraced by anesthesiologists, surgeons, and patients. The goal of the various techniques for continuous analgesia is to maintain the MEAC. This is accomplished by the administration of smaller doses of pain medication at more frequent intervals. In this way, the peaks and valleys of pain are smoothed out.

There are two basic methods of maintenance of an appropriate MEAC for an individual patient: patient-controlled analgesia (PCA) and continuous epidural analgesia.

Patient-Controlled Analgesia (PCA)

In PCA, a relatively new method, a programmable pump permits the patient to self-administer small intravenous doses of narcotics on demand as pain is felt. Therapeutic blood levels of narcotics can be maintained, and dosage can be tailored to the individual patient's needs. Inside the PCA machine is a syringe filled with narcotics (the "mechanical nurse"), a mechanism to drive the syringe, and digital electronics to program the amount of narcotic delivered when the patient presses a button. The machine is programmed to allow a minimum time interval between doses (the "lock-out interval"), which prevents the patient from overdosing. Security locks and alarms prevent tampering with the machine.

Your surgeon writes orders for the type of narcotic to be used, the initial loading dose (to bring you up to the therapeutic level), and the lock-out time. All you have to do is push the button when you want more pain relief. If you press the button too often, you trigger the lock-out feature and a record is made of your request, but no narcotic is given until the lock-out time has passed. If you need more pain relief than has been ordered and programmed into the PCA, speak to your surgeon, who can change the program.

Patient-controlled analgesia has been available in some U.S. hospitals since 1984, but it has only recently enjoyed widespread use. It has an excellent safety record, and you should ask about it when you speak to your anesthesiologist and surgeon prior to surgery.

Continuous Epidural Analgesia

In addition to its use as a method of anesthesia during surgery, epidural analgesia can be used by anesthesiologists for pain control after surgery. By injecting small, frequent amounts of opiates into the epidural space surrounding the spinal cord, your doctors can provide you with excellent pain relief.

In practice, however, it is somewhat more tricky to do than PCA. Since narcotics can diffuse from the epidural space to the brain by way of the spinal fluid, alterations in consciousness and possible depression of the cerebral centers of respiration may occur. This is not dangerous if it's recognized promptly, since a potent reversal agent, naloxone, is available and works almost immediately. Whereas naloxone rescue is necessary in only about 0.3 percent of cases, continuous epidural analgesia does require a high level of observation by trained personnel in order to ensure patient safety.

There are also a few side effects of epidural analgesia that occur in a small number of patients. These include a generalized rash and itching, an inability to urinate, dizziness when standing, and muscle weakness, making early walking difficult. So far, no studies have demonstrated that continuous epidural analgesia is more effective than patient-controlled analgesia, which presents fewer complications and fewer side effects. Either technique, however, is vastly superior to the old method of periodic intramuscular or intravenous administration of opiates.

"The Patch"

Considerable research is currently being done on pain control, and we are learning more about the mechanisms responsible for the sensation of pain. One area of interest is administration of narcotics directly through the skin. In its current form, this involves the slow, sustained release of a narcotic from a transdermal patch placed on the patient's skin.

Because it's more difficult to regulate MEAC from a transdermal patch, this approach to pain control so far seems less promising for short-term postoperative analgesia than it is for more chronic long-standing pain conditions.

11

YOUR OPERATION: BEFORE AND AFTER

Most people equate surgery with the actual operative procedure. Even though the technical performance of your operation is critical for overall success, surgery involves much more. A considerable amount of planning is required. Preoperative evaluation is necessary to ensure that the correct diagnosis has, in fact, been made, that an appropriate operative technique has been chosen, and that you're in good enough condition to withstand the physical demands that your operation will place on you.

SCHEDULING AND PREOPERATIVE TESTING

Once you have accepted the need for surgery, you will have to decide about the timing of your operation. If the condition is an emergency, requiring immediate admission to the hospital, you may have few if any options. But if your condition is not urgent, if it doesn't have a high potential for damage in a brief time, you may "elect" to have your operation at some more convenient future date. Many things may influence your decision: Job commitments, annual insurance deductibles, family considerations, holidays, the surgeon's schedule or the hospital's all may influence the choice of a specific date for your operation. But the term *elective* has more to do with "when" than with "whether" you'll have the operation. It doesn't usually imply that you can safely decide not to go ahead with the procedure.

For most operations performed today, preoperative testing, including a complete medical history and physical examination, is usually required. If your operation will involve being put to sleep, most hospitals require that studies be made of your heart, lungs, and kidneys by means of an electrocardiogram (EKG), chest X ray, and urinalysis. Blood tests are also required to check for infection, blood clotting abnormalities, or any other conditions that might make surgery difficult, if not impossible.

Preoperative testing is often done several days before the operation itself. This may be inconvenient, since it requires a separate trip to the hospital, but often it can be carried out by your primary-care physician at his or her own office, who will then send the report to the surgeon or the hospital.

If any of the screening tests reveal an abnormality, your doctor may ask for additional tests or a consultation with other medical specialists. If serious coexisting conditions are found, consultants may be required to correct those problems before surgery can be performed. Sometimes, obtaining medical clearance may delay the date of surgery. If that happens to you, keep in mind that it's in your best interest to obtain as much information as possible about your general condition and any increased surgical risk prior to your operation. Treating a preexisting condition will usually improve your chances for successful surgery. Even if a condition is discovered but cannot be effectively treated, simply knowing of its existence can change the way an operation is performed, or how postoperative care is managed. For example, discovering significant heart disease in a patient about to undergo major blood-vessel surgery can materially affect the surgeon's choice of an operative procedure and the selection of materials used to repair the vessel, as well as signaling the need for heightened postoperative heart monitoring in an intensive care unit rather than on the ward.

Today, many surgical procedures are performed without actual hospital admission, as "same-day," "walk-in," or "ambulatory" surgery. With this type of surgery, it's best if you arrange to have someone take you home afterward, since you may feel unsteady from your anesthesia or pain medications.

Even for patients whose operation requires a night or more in the hospital (inpatient surgery), many insurance companies currently refuse to pay for any hospital days before the day of surgery. This is done in an effort to reduce the costs of hospitalization, but it means that you will be admitted on the day of surgery (same-day admission). Of course, this also means that your preoperative testing will have to be done on a separate visit in order to be ready by the time of the proposed operation. In general, you should view preoperative testing, as inconvenient as it may be, as another type of medical insurance—insurance that you're in the best possible shape so that your surgery will go smoothly.

BLOOD TRANSFUSION

If your surgeon tells you that your operation may require a blood transfusion, a number of concerns may be raised. Today, most hospitals stock emergency supplies of virtually all blood types. What they don't have they can quickly get from a regional blood bank. Donated blood is subjected to several levels of screening for contamination, ranging from detailed questionnaires and interviews to an array of sophisticated laboratory tests. Transfusion therapy is now one of the safest of all major medical treatments.

Nevertheless, many people remain wary of the blood supply. The main reason, of course, is fear of AIDS, but the risk of becoming infected with the AIDS virus through a blood transfusion is now extremely remote. According to recent estimates, 1 in every 165,000 to 225,000 units (pints) of blood is contaminated with the virus. (The average transfusion patient receives a total of about two and a half units of blood.) The risk of getting hepatitis from a blood transfusion is much higher, but still relatively slim: About 1 in every 330 units carries the disease.

Some patients request donations from close friends or relatives rather than turn to the public blood supply. But that's not necessarily a safer bet—and may, in fact, be less safe. That's because such "directed donations" bypass one of the most important safeguards in blood banking—anonymity. Someone who donates blood anonymously has no incentive (since donors are no longer paid) to disguise the fact that he or she may be in a high-risk group for transmitting disease. A friend or relative, on the other hand, might be reluctant to disclose how he or she happens to fall into one of those high-risk groups.

So although there's some risk of infection from the public blood supply, that risk is relatively insignificant in a life-or-death emergency. However, only about 20 percent of all transfusions are used for emergencies: Most of the rest go to nonemergency surgical procedures.

Many patients scheduled for elective operations use the public blood supply unnecessarily. They could eliminate the risk of infection altogether, and help conserve the public supply for emergency use, by donating blood to themselves instead. The procedure is simple: You donate as often as once a week beginning a month or so before your scheduled surgery. Your physician monitors your blood count and gives you iron supplements as needed to ensure that nothing more than a mild anemia develops.

Most insurance companies will cover the cost of autologous transfusions, as they are called, as long as you're storing blood for upcoming surgery at your physician's request. Note, however, that insurance coverage applies only to blood that's actually transfused, not to units donated beyond what you need. If you're facing surgery that might require blood, discuss autologous transfusions with your surgeon.

ADMISSION

Since your doctor has already informed the hospital you are coming, they are expecting you. However, a little planning on your part can make hospital admission less burdensome. Remember to bring your insurance card and any personal articles—toothbrush, robe, slippers—that you think you'll need. But if you forget anything, such personal items are for sale in most hospitals.

When you get to the hospital, you go to the admissions department, where your insurance will be verified, a name tag will be applied to your wrist, and a room assigned. You should know that most insurance policies do not pay for a private room, so if you want to have that degree of privacy, you'll probably be responsible for the difference in rates between a semiprivate and a private room. In some hospitals, this could amount to $200 a day and up. If you're in doubt about your insurance policy, ask the admissions clerk for help.

"Living Wills"

While you're in the admissions area, ask about a living will if the admissions clerk does not raise the subject with you. Living wills, now known as advance medical directives (AMDs), are standardized documents that permit you to tell your doctors how you want to be treated when you can no longer speak for yourself. If a major postoperative complication such as a stroke should leave you unable to communicate, this document would permit your doctors to follow your desires regarding artificial means of life support or the administration of certain medicines if a panel of other physicians concluded that your situation was hopeless.

In 1990 the U.S. Supreme Court endorsed the use of these directives. They seemed like an effective way to avoid a dreaded fate: being subjected to treatments that prolong life, sometimes indefinitely and at great expense, when there's no hope of recovering from a grave condition. Unfortunately, recent studies have shown that AMDs have had little impact on the way people are actually treated at the end of their life. Often, doctors who are given such a document don't follow its instructions. That may be because the document tries to cover all possible situations with a broad statement such as "I do not want life-sustaining treatment if I am dying or permanently unconscious." But it's often unclear how such statements apply to specific situations. Does "life-sustaining" therapy, for example, mean only mechanical breathing and artificial feeding, or does it extend to giving antibiotics or amputating an infected leg? And general statements don't allow people to specify different wishes for a variety of different situations. In a 1993 study of 150 California physicians, the proportion of doctors who said they would follow an advance directive and refrain from treating a patient jumped from 55 to 71 percent when they saw a specific directive rather than a general one.

Even when doctors have a clear guide to a person's wishes, they may not follow them, in part because they're unfamiliar with the law. According to decisions by the U.S. Supreme Court and several lower courts, patients have a right to refuse treatment, and doctors can honor such requests with no risk of liability. But in a California study, three fourths of the physicians said they would refuse to disconnect a tube supplying food and water to someone in an apparently irreversible coma, and one third would not unplug a breathing machine—even when a patient's advance directive explicitly forbade life-sustaining treatment in that situation. Another recent study, involving nearly 700 physicians, confirmed that many doctors don't know the requirements of the law. And others may find it difficult to forgo treatment simply because they've been trained to keep patients alive at all costs.

So it's important to be specific. To avoid vague generalities, a new form for an advance medical directive has been developed. It permits you to make specific choices about a variety of procedures under six different circumstances. You can get a copy of that form by sending a stamped self-addressed envelope to Consumer Reports on Health, Department AD, 101 Truman Avenue, Yonkers, NY 10703-1057.

But even that may not be enough. It's essential to attach that document to a completed copy of the standard advance directive for your state. While such standard directives are not very specific, doctors are more likely to recognize the state form itself as a legal document. You may be able to get a copy of your state form from a local hospital or from the state health department. Or you can write to Choice in Dying—a not-for-profit organization that distributes free copies of the state documents—at 200 Varick Street, New York, NY 10014.

Even the most detailed directive cannot possibly anticipate every situation that may arise. And doctors may interpret your written wishes in ways you didn't intend. That's why it's also important to appoint a family member or close friend to act as your agent, or proxy, by making out a form known as either a durable power of attorney for health care or a health-care proxy. If you become unable to communicate, the agent decides, based on your written instructions and his or her personal knowledge of your preferences, what course of action you would choose. Such proxy decision making, which has been endorsed by the Supreme Court, can reassure a hesitant doctor that a particular course really does represent your wishes.

You can minimize the chance that your doctor or your agent will misinterpret or ignore your wishes by discussing what you want in detail with both of them. Going over the twelve situations described in the form will give them a clearer sense of how much you'd be willing to endure to preserve your life. The discussion also lets you find out ahead of time whether your physician and your agent would be willing to go along with your wishes, particularly in the situation where doctors as well as proxies often hesitate to act, such as unplugging a life-support machine or cutting off artificial feeding. If your doctor or agent questions your right to refuse any treatment, you might ask him or her to check with an attorney who knows the law on advance directives but doesn't work for a hospital. (Hospital lawyers may give overly cautious advice designed mainly to protect the hospital.) If the doctor's or agent's reservations persist, consider looking for someone more willing to comply with your wishes.

Of course, none of these steps will do any good unless your doctor and your agent get copies of your advance directive. Don't leave it in your safe-deposit box! Distribute several copies, not only to your doctor and your agent, but also to your lawyer and to immediate family members or a close friend.

CHECKING IN

When you leave the admissions area, you will be escorted to your designated room. There you will meet the nurses assigned to your case. If you have not already done so, now is a good time to give all of your valuables to a family member to take home. Better still, don't bring jewelry or other valuables to the hospital. Simply put, things disappear.

Soon, your doctor or an associate will arrive to take a history of your illness and perform a physical examination, if that has not already been done. More laboratory work may be required. If any special preparations for your operation are necessary, such as medications, enemas, or shaving, they will be done now. Unless your doctor has ordered a special diet, you'll be given regular hospital food. A staff dietitian may visit you to discuss your preferences or requirements. So if you have allergies or strong likes and dislikes regarding food, be sure to make them known.

A representative from the anesthesia department will come to see you to evaluate your risk for general or spinal anesthesia, if that is what has been chosen (see Chapter 10). This is your opportunity to ask questions and make all your wishes about anesthesia known.

SURVIVING A HOSPITAL STAY

Hospitals work best for you when you ask for what you want. Seldom will hospital staffers come into your room and ask what they can do for you. Make your wishes known. Obviously, your doctor won't necessarily agree with everything you want, since some of your requests might not be compatible with good medical care, but at least you can ask. The important thing is not to be afraid to ask questions and make requests.

According to a recent study, nearly 1 out of every 25 patients is actually injured during his or her hospital stay. Whereas most of those injuries result from unavoidable risks of therapy, more than a quarter stem from mistakes made by the hospital staff. In addition to outright mistakes, many patients experience unnecessary discomfort and inconvenience in a hospital. But there are ways to protect yourself and to get the attention you need.

Among the most common hospital mistakes are giving patients the wrong drug dose and giving a medication, test, or procedure meant for someone else. To spot such errors, you have to know what drugs or procedures should be coming your way. That means staying alert and asking the right questions. If you're too sick for that, have a family member or close friend act on your behalf.

Your drug regimen in the hospital may be different from the one you followed at home. Medications may be dropped or added. The times you take them may differ, too. Ask your doctor to explain any changes. Before you take any new drug, make sure the nurse checks to be sure the medication is for you. Then ask for the name of the drug and note its appearance. If those don't jibe with what your doctor said you'd be getting, ask the nurse to check the order book or contact your physician.

You should be informed about the purpose, risks, and discomfort of any test or procedure you'll be undergoing. You should also know about special pretest preparations, such as laxatives and enemas before intestinal X rays, or fasting before stomach X rays. Knowing what to expect may also help in case the food service mistakenly sends up a meal just before a test that requires an empty stomach.

Many hospitals, especially in large cities, face a shortage of funds. As a result, some hospitals may provide less individualized service. Tasteless food, delayed responses by nurses and aides, curt replies from overworked staff, and inconveniently scheduled tests are practically inevitable. But you can usually get your important needs met, if you know when and how to ask.

Pressing the call button for minor matters too frequently can convince the nursing staff that you're a chronic malcontent. (It's sad but true that incidents that truly bother patients may seem "minor" to hospital staff.) But that doesn't mean you should keep quiet about problems. If the food is not just tasteless but consistently burned, undercooked, or cold, you have every right to complain. If talking to the nurse doesn't help, call the dietitian. If you're exhausted because nurses awaken you in the middle of the night for medications or routine checks, ask your doctor whether your drug schedule can be rearranged or whether that 4:00 A.M. blood-pressure check is absolutely necessary.

Sometimes it's worth doing more than just asking, even if you risk raising some hackles. You don't have to tolerate rudeness. You shouldn't have to put up with hour-long waits for necessary assistance. If your nurse consistently ignores your reasonable requests, speak to the head nurse and, if necessary, to the nursing supervisor or your doctor.

In addition, many hospitals employ specially trained patient advocates. Their job is to listen to your complaint and intercede for you with the hospital staff. If you're getting nowhere with the staff, contact the advocate.

KNOW YOUR RIGHTS

The Patient's Bill of Rights, drawn up by the American Hospital Association in 1973, specifies your rights as a hospital patient. You should receive a copy when you're admitted. If you're well enough, be sure to read it. Here are three of your most important rights:

- To receive complete, understandable information about your diagnosis, treatment, and expected outcome.

- To review your medical record. Such records can be difficult to decipher. Ask your physician about anything you can't make out.
- To refuse any treatment or test. Unless you're unconscious or require emergency care, every procedure requires consent. And major procedures require informed consent. That means doctors must explain the benefits and risks to your satisfaction before you sign on the dotted line.

To obtain a copy of the complete Patient's Bill of Rights, contact either the patient advocate or the admissions office at your local hospital.

THE DAY OF SURGERY AND BEYOND

On the day of your operation, you may receive some medications to make the introduction of anesthesia easier and safer. These agents will also have the effect of making you relaxed and drowsy. If you are an inpatient, the orderly will come with a gurney (a stretcher on wheels) to transport you to the operating room area. Usually, you will go to a preoperative holding area first, where an anesthesiologist will speak with you and start an intravenous drip of fluids. If your anesthesiologist or surgeon requires any specialized tubes, such as a pulmonary artery catheter or an arterial line, these may be placed at this time. All of your records and laboratory results will be checked again.

When it's time for your operation, you will be transported to the operating suite itself. In the operating room, you will be placed on a narrow table. (If you feel cold, say so and ask for blankets.) As you look around, you will see operating lights above you and large anesthesia machines at the head of your table. A scrub nurse (already gowned and gloved) presides over a large table covered with surgical instruments; he or she hands the surgeon the instruments and sutures required to perform your operation. Another nurse, called a "circulating nurse," is present to help you and to obtain any required items that may not be present in the room. Usually your surgeon or the surgical assistant is also present at this time.

If you are having general anesthesia, the anesthesiologist will place an oxygen mask over your nose and mouth and ask you to breath deeply. You will then be given an intravenous sedative. Following this injection, you will remember nothing and awaken after the operation is completed.

Once you're asleep, an endotracheal tube will be placed in your windpipe through your mouth to more effectively control the administration of the anesthetic gases. Any other tubes which you might need, and whose insertion might cause you discomfort if you were awake, such as a Foley catheter into the bladder or a nasogastric tube into the stomach, are passed at this time. The surgeon and assistant surgeon will then apply an antiseptic solution to the site of the proposed operation and apply sterile drapes to cover all of your body except for the surgical site. Your operation is then performed.

When the operation has been completed, a dressing is applied and the level of anesthetic gas is gradually reduced. When you are breathing on your own without assistance, you are transported from the operating room to a recovery area. Here you will be closely monitored until the effects of the anesthesia have worn off. It is here that most patients awaken and begin to experience pain. When you are fully awake, you will again be transferred, this time back to your room or, if your condition warrants, to a more specialized monitoring center called an "intensive care unit."

Recovery following a surgical procedure is variable, being influenced by the severity of the underlying disease, the presence of any other diseases or disorders, the difficulty of the operation, and the development of any complications. You can materially affect your recovery from surgery by eliminating those complications that are in your power to control. Two of the most important things you can do are to cough and to walk whenever you are asked to do so. Coughing helps prevent postoperative pneumonia, and walking helps prevent clots from forming in your veins. Such clots may migrate from leg veins to the lungs, causing pulmonary emboli, which in certain instances can be fatal. Early ambulation after surgery is indeed an ounce of prevention.

As your surgeon should explain *before* the operation, you may awake from anesthesia to discover various tubes coming from your body. The endotracheal tube may be left in place for a short while if your doctors believe that its presence will enable you to breathe more easily. Since it passes through your larynx, you won't be able to speak until it is removed. If you have had an abdominal operation, you may have a nasogastric (NG) tube coming from your stomach through your nose. This is to keep your stomach empty and keep you from vomiting and possibly drawing gastric contents into the windpipe. The NG tube will be removed as soon as normal function returns to your intestines (usually two to five days). There may be a tube in your bladder (a Foley catheter) to drain urine; this tube is usually removed when you are alert and moving about.

Your surgeon may have placed other tubes designed to drain various body fluids, which are removed only after their usefulness has ended. In general, you can always tell when you're getting better after surgery: People keep taking out your tubes.

You may also be hooked up to continuous monitoring instruments, such as an electrocardiograph or gauges to measure central venous pressure, arterial pressure, pulmonary capillary pressure, and oxygen saturation. Each is designed to provide moment-to-moment information of your body's response to the stress of surgery. As you improve, the monitors are discontinued.

When you have inhalation anesthesia or spinal anesthesia, all body processes are slowed, including intestinal function. This is why food intake is limited for several days after major surgery; it takes more time for the intestine to "awaken" than it does for the brain. Wait until you get home to try a pizza.

One of the most important aspects of your operation, pain control, is discussed in Chapter 10.

Long-term recovery and the ability to return to one's normal lifestyle vary markedly among patients, even for the same conditions and following the same operations. The wisest course here is to thoroughly question your surgeon about when you can resume eating certain foods or exercising, when you can return to work, or any other concerns that you might have. Many patients find it convenient to make a list of their questions so that nothing will be forgotten. You should consider the answers to these questions as part of your surgeon's service to you. Since it's important, and you have already paid for it, make sure you don't leave the hospital without it!

Checklist for Your Operation

1. Informed consent

Have all options been explained?

Have you understood all risks and benefits?

2. Scheduling of elective surgery

Insurance deductible?

Okay with employer?

3. Preoperative procedures

Have you or your primary-care physician told your surgeon about all your preexisting medical conditions?

Has all necessary lab work been done?

Is autologous transfusion necessary?

4. What to bring to the hospital

Your insurance card

A copy of your living will

Pajamas, robe, slippers, personal toilet articles

No valuables

5. Surgical concerns

Have you discussed your choice of anesthesia?

Do you want a sleeping pill the night before surgery?

Has your surgeon told you about your likely postoperative condition?

6. Before you go home

Have you made a list of all your questions about aftercare so you can get complete instructions from your surgeon?

12

OPERATIONS AND OBSERVATIONS

This chapter provides information regarding the surgical procedures most commonly performed in the United States today.

Each entry indicates the purpose of or indications for the surgery; discusses the nonsurgical alternatives, if any; describes the surgical technique and the preferred anesthesia; discusses any risks or complications; and describes the typical postoperative course.

Table 12.1 lists the 34 most common operations performed in the hospital setting.

TABLE 12.1

The Most Common Inpatient Surgical Procedures in the United States (1992)

1. Obstetrical Procedures		6,664,000
Episiotomy	1,611,000	
Cesarean section	921,000	
2. Gastrointestinal Procedures		5,358,000
Endoscopy	1,437,000	
Cholecystectomy	525,000	
Lysis of adhesions	344,000	
Appendectomy	261,000	
Colectomy	217,000	
Inguinal herniorrhaphy	139,000	
3. Cardiovascular Procedures		4,424,000
Cardiac catheterization	1,028,000	
Coronary artery bypass graft	468,000	
Pacemaker implantation	274,000	
Blood vessel surgery	178,000	
4. Musculoskeletal Procedures		3,266,000
Arthroscopy	534,000	
Open reduction, internal fixation	417,000	
Laminectomy and spine fusion	319,000	
Arthroplasty	394,000	
5. Gynecological Surgery		2,302,000
Hysterectomy	580,000	
Salpingo-oophorectomy	464,000	
Tubal ligation/destruction	380,000	
Dilation and curettage	173,000	
Repair of pelvic hernias	141,000	

6. Genitourinary Procedures		1,942,000
Cystoscopy	414,000	
Prostatectomy	353,000	
7. Skin Surgery		1,371,000
Skin biopsy	1,065,000	
Skin graft	108,000	
8. Breast Surgery		540,000
Mastectomy	170,000	
Lumpectomy	45,000	
Simple mastectomy	12,000	
Modified radical mastectomy	97,000	
9. Thoracic Surgery		1,030,000
Bronchoscopy	315,000	
Pulmonary resection	208,000	
10. Central Nervous System Surgery		921,000
Craniotomy	202,000	
11. Eye Surgery		332,000
Cataract extraction	197,000	

Source: National Center for Health Care Statistics
Note: Since only the most common surgical procedures are covered here, the total number of operations in a category may be larger than the sum of the listed procedures.

OBSTETRICAL PROCEDURES

Episiotomy (Enlarging the vaginal opening)

1. Purpose of the Procedure: To prevent uncontrolled tearing of the vagina and rectum during childbirth. Most often necessary during a woman's first delivery, in premature labor, when the baby is unusually large, or when a forceps delivery is required.

2. Nonsurgical Alternatives: Certain maneuvers, such as predelivery perineal exercise and vertical (squatting) delivery positions, may reduce the need for episiotomy. But since the procedure is largely preventive, the obstetrician's clinical judgment determines the necessity in each case.

3. Anesthesia: Whatever anesthesia is being used for the delivery itself (epidural, caudal, etc.). If no anesthesia has been given, episiotomy may be done with local anesthesia.

4. Surgical Technique: The incision is usually made at the back of the vaginal opening and may extend to one side in order to avoid injuring the anal sphincter. Following delivery, the tissues that were cut are repaired with absorbable stitches.

5. Risks: Bleeding and infection rarely occur.

6. What to Expect: Pain or soreness may last a few weeks. Sitting in a warm bath helps the discomfort. Any drainage should be brought to the doctor's attention. Intercourse should not be resumed until after the doctor's six-week postpartum examination indicates that healing is complete.

Cesarean Section (Surgical abdominal delivery)

1. Purpose of the Procedure: To avoid or reduce the risk when vaginal delivery is difficult, complicated, or impossible. Causes include premature delivery, breech or other abnormal presentation, disproportion between the

size of the baby's head and the mother's pelvis, protracted labor, fetal distress, or maternal exhaustion.

2. Nonsurgical Alternatives: Vaginal delivery is the obvious, "natural" alternative. Cesareans should usually be chosen as a method of delivery only after failure of a trial of labor. Many women who have had C-sections in the past can safely deliver through the normal birth canal (called "VBAC"—vaginal birth after Cesarean), so previous C-section is only sometimes an indication.

3. Anesthesia: Epidural, spinal, or general

4. Surgical Technique: An incision is made into the lower abdomen, followed by an incision into the uterus. The baby is removed from the womb, the placenta is removed, and the incision is sutured closed. (If no further pregnancies are desired, tubal ligation—tying off of the Fallopian tubes—can be carried out before the abdomen is closed.)

5. Risks:

a. To the mother, small risk of wound, bladder, or kidney infection. Small risk of hemorrhage.

b. To the infant, the risk is variable and dependent upon the specific reason for the C-section.

6. What to Expect:

a. Postpartum bleeding from the vagina (lochia) for four to eight weeks, as after normal delivery.

b. Wound pain for about a week.

c. Length of hospital stay: four to seven days.

d. Return to normal activity: four to six weeks.

GASTROINTESTINAL PROCEDURES

Endoscopy (Internal examination of the intestine)

1. Purpose of the Procedure:

a. To examine the lining of the gastrointestinal tract.

b. To remove a small tissue sample for diagnosis by microscopic examination (biopsy).

c. To treat abnormalities not requiring open surgery, such as polyps.

2. Nonsurgical Alternatives: In many cases, X-ray studies of the esophagus, stomach, and small bowel (barium swallow) or of the rectum, colon, and ileum (barium enema) should precede endoscopy, as they are less expensive and may obviate the need for endoscopy.

3. Anesthesia: Local anesthetic sprayed into the mouth and throat (for upper intestinal endoscopy), supplemented with intravenous sedative drugs.

4. Surgical Technique: A flexible hollow tube with a fiberoptic miniaturized video camera is introduced into the mouth for examination of the esophagus (esophagoscopy), stomach (gastroscopy), small bowel (duodenoscopy), pancreas (pancreatography); or into the rectum for examination of the large bowel (colonoscopy). Instruments passed through the endoscope permit the operator to take small pieces of tissue (biopsies) for diagnosis by microscopic examination. Similar techniques can be used to insert feeding tubes into the stomach through the abdominal wall (gastrostomy) or into the small bowel (feeding jejunostomy) for purposes of long-term feeding, whenever food cannot be taken by mouth.

With a procedure called "endoscopic cholangiopancreatography," or ERCP, the drainage system of the liver and the pancreas can be examined by injecting a substance that shows up on X rays.

5. Risks: Complications are extremely rare for most diagnostic procedures, but there is a 2 to 3 percent risk of pancreatitis with ERCP. When endoscopy is used for therapy, risk of bleeding, perforation, or infection varies with the condition being treated.

6. What to Expect:

a. Endoscopy is usually performed as an outpatient procedure, often in a physician's office.

b. Preparation involves fasting on the morning of the test, along with laxatives or enemas if colonoscopy is planned.

c. Some discomfort during the procedure.

d. Fatigue, dizziness, or nausea following sedation. Have someone available to drive you home.

e. Sore throat for one or two days following esophagoscopy.

f. Flatulence or bloating for several hours.

Cholecystectomy (Removal of the gallbladder)

1. Purpose of the Procedure:

a. To relieve acute or chronic abdominal pain associated with gallstones.

b. To treat gallbladder disease and its complications, such as jaundice or pancreatitis.

2. Nonsurgical Alternatives: Patients with gallstones that are uncomplicated and asymptomatic do not require treatment.

Several new nonsurgical therapies are now used to reduce the size of symptomatic gallstones enough to let them pass spontaneously into the intestine. But half of all patients successfully treated without surgery will form new stones within five years unless gallstone-dissolving drugs are taken continuously.

a. Gallstone-dissolving drugs, such as ursodiol, may be tried as initial therapy. They cause stones to dissolve, but slowly. Treatment takes anywhere from six months to two years, at $4 to $6 per day for the drugs. Patients must have a functioning gallbladder and noncalcium-containing stones smaller than a half inch in diameter. The drugs may adversely affect liver function, and the long-term side effects remain uncertain. Only one patient in five with gallstones is a suitable candidate for this drug.

b. Lithotripsy (literally "rock crushing") may be used alone or in combination with oral drugs. The patient is sedated or anesthetized and immersed in a water bath or positioned behind a water-filled cushion. A shock wave aimed at the gallbladder passes through the water and breaks up the stones, allowing them to pass into the intestine. Since patients must have a functioning gallbladder and no more than three stones, none larger than one inch in diameter, fewer than 2 patients in 10 with gallstones are candidates for this approach. Patients often report abdominal pain in the weeks or months following treatment as stone fragments continue to pass. Long-term therapy with ursodiol is necessary to prevent reformation of gallstones.

3. Anesthesia: General

4. Surgical Techniques: The gallbladder can be removed either through a traditional surgical incision or by using the newer laparoscopic, or "pinhole," approach. In the traditional "open" technique, a long incision severs abdominal muscles and nerves, and therefore results in

greater postoperative pain and restriction of activity than does the pinhole approach. Compared with the laparoscopic approach, however, the open technique provides markedly better surgical exposure, with considerably less risk of injury to the common bile duct, an important conduit of bile from the liver to the intestine. Such an injury is rarely fatal, but it is serious and requires complicated corrective surgery.

Today, open gallbladder surgery is usually performed only when conditions are not favorable for the laparoscopic approach. Those conditions include extensive intra-abdominal scarring, large stones in the common bile duct, pregnancy beyond the sixth month, and severe inflammation of the pancreas.

Laparoscopic cholecystectomy requires only three or four small abdominal incisions, each about a quarter to a half inch long. Specially designed instruments and the laparoscope, a narrow lighted tube with a miniature video camera, are inserted through the incisions. Guided by a video monitor, the surgeon detaches the gallbladder and removes it through one of the incisions. There's less pain, less scarring, and a shorter hospital stay than with the open approach.

5. Risks: Common-duct injuries are very rare after cholecystectomy by either approach, but they occur more commonly after laparoscopic cholecystectomy. The frequency of this complication decreases when a surgeon has performed more than 100 laparoscopic cholecystectomies. For this reason, make sure your surgeon has performed at least that number of laparoscopic procedures on the gallbladder.

The mortality rate for either approach—open or laparoscopic—is low, only 0.3 percent.

In about 10 percent of cases, unexpected scar tissue, an obstructed view, internal bleeding, or some other factor forces the surgeon to convert to open abdominal surgery midway through the laparoscopic procedure.

6. What to Expect: When performed for proper indications, cholecystectomy relieves symptoms in 85 percent of patients.

Postoperative recovery from laparoscopic cholecystectomy is usually quite rapid, often less than one week before patients resume work and exercise. Some patients experience flatulence or loose stools after eating fats. This usually improves over several months.

All other things being equal, choose the laparoscopic approach, but be sure to select a surgeon with sufficient training and clinical experience in laparoscopic technique.

Lysis of Adhesions (Removal of intestinal scar tissue)

1. Purpose of the Procedure: To relieve complete or partial obstruction of the small intestine or colon due to kinking of the bowel caused by contraction of intra-abdominal scar tissue (adhesions). Adhesions develop in all patients following any type of abdominal surgery, but they can also be caused by any intra-abdominal inflammatory reaction. Only 2 percent are ever severe enough to result in obstruction of the intestine. Adhesions may cause abdominal distention, pain, cramping, vomiting, and inability to pass feces or intestinal gas.

2. Nonsurgical Treatment: Decompression of the gas-filled intestine can be tried by applying suction to a tube placed through the nose into the stomach or through the anus into the large bowel, depending on the site of

obstruction. This is not often successful in cases of complete obstruction.

3. Anesthesia: General

4. Surgical Technique: An incision is made in the abdomen large enough to permit exploration of the suspected area of obstruction. Once the scar tissue is found, it is cut and the areas of kinking are straightened, relieving the obstruction. Some surgeons now perform this operation laparoscopically, particularly in patients with partial intestinal obstruction.

5. Risks:

a. Since surgery for complete obstruction is usually performed as an emergency procedure (less than 24 hours after admission), mortality rates (5 percent) are higher than for elective surgery. If intestinal gangrene or perforation has developed prior to surgery, the mortality rate increases sixfold.

b. Once adhesions have resulted in intestinal obstruction and the necessity for surgery, future bouts of obstruction may be expected in as many as 30 percent of patients as more adhesions form.

6. What to Expect:

a. Hospital stay varies, usually from 5 to 10 days.

b. Normal diet is resumed during hospital stay.

c. Return to normal activity in three to four weeks.

Appendectomy (Removal of the appendix)

1. Purpose of the Procedure:

a. To remove an acutely inflamed or ruptured appendix; relieve the symptoms of acute appendicitis, such as abdominal pain, loss of appetite, nausea, vomiting, and low-grade fever; and prevent the spread of infection into the abdominal cavity and bloodstream.

b. To remove a healthy appendix in the course of other abdominal surgery, to prevent any future appendicitis. (Not advisable for persons over age 55, since the risk of the preventive surgery exceeds the risk of appendicitis.)

c. To remove a ruptured appendix after drainage of an appendiceal abscess—"interval appendectomy."

2. Nonsurgical Alternatives: None. Failure to treat appendicitis may result in rupture of the appendix, spreading infection throughout the abdominal cavity. Any abdominal pain lasting more than six hours, particularly if located in the lower right abdomen, should be suspected of being acute appendicitis.

3. Technique: Appendectomy, one of the most successful operations in all of surgery, is commonly performed through a small incision in the lower right side of the abdomen. It is sometimes necessary to leave a drain in for a few days after surgery. Some surgeons now perform appendectomies laparoscopically, citing shorter hospital stays and more rapid recovery.

4. Anesthesia: General

5. Risks: Mortality rate for uncomplicated acute appendicitis is 0.1 percent, but it can rise a hundredfold if the appendix ruptures. Since rupture of an acutely inflamed appendix usually occurs 24 hours or more after the onset of abdominal pain, medical attention should be sought prior to that time.

6. What to Expect:

a. Uncomplicated postoperative course includes a return to a light, semisolid diet within a day or two and discharge from the hospital in about three days. Walking and light activity are encouraged, but the patient should limit stair-climbing and heavy lifting for a few weeks. Stitches are removed after a week, and normal activity can be resumed after about three weeks.

b. Postoperative fever may signal the development of a wound infection or an abdominal abscess. Fever or diarrhea may point to an intestinal infection with an organism known as *C. difficile*. This sometimes occurs with the use of antibiotics.

c. High fever, chills, and increasing pain may indicate peritonitis, a potentially dangerous infection of the lining of the abdomen.

Colectomy (Removal of the colon)

1. Purpose of the Procedure:

a. Usually to treat cancer, diverticulitis, or inflammatory bowel disease (Crohn's disease, ulcerative colitis).

b. Less commonly, to treat volvulus (twisting), perforation, injuries, etc.

2. Nonsurgical Alternatives:

a. None for cancer.

b. For inflammatory bowel disease, a prolonged course of medical management is preferable to surgery, which is usually reserved for patients with complications, such as bleeding, perforation, obstruction, or failure of medical management.

3. Anesthesia: General

4. Surgical Technique: The vast majority of colon operations are still performed by conventional surgery, using standard vertical or transverse abdominal incisions.

A segment of the colon is removed and the ends are then rejoined, if possible. If not, the upper end is brought to the surface of the abdomen creating a temporary or permanent opening (colostomy) for the excretion of intestinal contents into an attached bag.

Laparoscopic techniques have recently been used with increasing success to avoid large abdominal incisions. The need for a temporary colostomy has been decreasing in recent years because of technical improvements, such as the intestinal stapling device, which rejoins the intestine without the necessity for sutures.

5. Risks:

a. Overall mortality risk is 2 percent, resulting from intestinal contents leaking from the site where the colon was reconnected (the anastomosis).

b. If leakage occurs, reoperation may be necessary.

6. What to Expect:

a. Hospital stay: one to two weeks.

b. If a temporary colostomy is necessary, it can usually be closed at a second operation one to two months later.

c. If a large part of the colon is removed, bowel movements may increase in frequency, occurring up to six to eight times a day. In time, with appropriate medication, this can almost always be reduced to two to three times a day.

d. In the absence of complications, full recovery can be anticipated in six to eight weeks.

Inguinal Herniorrhaphy (Repair of groin hernia)

1. Purpose of the Procedure: To correct an abnormal protrusion of the intestine through a part of the abdominal wall.

2. Nonsurgical Alternatives: A truss can be worn under the clothing to keep the hernia from growing worse until surgery can be scheduled, but that is not recommended as a permanent solution. Failure to repair a groin hernia exposes the patient to at least a 5 percent risk of intestinal obstruction and gangrene caused by the hernia.

3. Anesthesia: General, spinal, epidural, or local

4. Surgical Techniques:

a. In open herniorrhaphy: a standard surgical incision is made and the protruding section of intestine is pushed back into the abdominal cavity. The surrounding tissues are closed with sutures to obliterate the abnormal opening in the abdominal wall.

b. In laparoscopic herniorrhaphy: an internal layer of synthetic mesh is placed over the defect in the abdominal wall.

5. Risks:

a. Currently, it appears that the failure rate is slightly higher with the laparoscopic technique (3 to 5 percent compared with 1 to 2 percent for the open procedure). Balancing the increased risk of recurrence is the shortened recovery time and less initial discomfort. As with laparoscopic gallbladder surgery, it's wise to make sure your surgeon has had extensive experience (more than 50 cases).

b. Other risks—urinary retention and wound infection—are rare.

6. What to Expect:

a. Hospital stays of one to two days are uncommon. Most surgeons now perform herniorrhaphy as an outpatient procedure.

b. Full activity can be resumed in six to eight weeks.
c. Discomfort in the groin rarely persists for longer than a month or two after successful hernia repair.
d. Recurrence of the hernia, signaled by pain or the formation of a lump at the site of the original repair, occurs in fewer than 5 percent of cases.

CARDIOVASCULAR PROCEDURES

Cardiac Catheterization (Examination of the heart, its chambers, and its arteries)

1. Purpose of the Procedure:
a. To evaluate the condition and function of the heart and its valves, chambers, and blood vessels.
b. To unclog a narrowed coronary artery (coronary angioplasty).

2. Nonsurgical Alternatives: In general, cardiac catheterization is not attempted unless nonsurgical procedures, such as electrocardiography, cardiac sonography (ultrasound), thallium scanning (specialized X-ray studies), or stress testing have proved inconclusive or have indicated that further testing is necessary.

3. Anesthesia: Local with sedation

4. Technique: A needle puncture is made over a blood vessel, usually in the groin but sometimes in the arm or neck. The catheter, a long, hollow plastic tube of small diameter, is inserted into the blood vessel and then advanced into the heart under X-ray guidance. Blood pressure can be measured, blood samples can be withdrawn through the catheter, and pictures of the inside

of the heart and its blood vessels (the coronary arteries) can be obtained by injecting a contrast material that shows up on X rays (coronary arteriography).

5. Risks: Catheterization of the heart may cause irregular heartbeats, blood clots, and allergic reactions. In the case of fewer than 1 percent of coronary arteriography patients, the procedure may actually precipitate a heart attack.

6. What to Expect:

a. Patients typically experience 20 to 30 seconds of a hot sensation, or "flushing," during the injection of the X-ray dye.

b. The site at which the catheter was inserted requires firm pressure, then careful observation for 8 to 24 hours, since bleeding from the vessel is a complication in 1 to 2 percent of cases.

Coronary Artery Bypass Graft

1. Purpose of the Procedure:

a. To increase the supply of blood to the heart muscle and thus relieve the symptoms of coronary artery disease, primarily angina pectoris (chest pain).

b. As an emergency treatment, to restore blood supply to the heart in a severe heart attack (myocardial infarction).

2. Nonsurgical Alternatives:

a. Since coronary artery bypass grafting does not usually prolong a patient's life or even reliably prevent future heart attacks, medical therapy is often a good alternative. Many patients experience a marked improvement in symptoms and lifestyle on a closely monitored regime of medication, diet, and exercise.

b. In patients with disease limited essentially to one or two coronary arteries, balloon angioplasty can be attempted. This is a technique for reopening a narrowed coronary-artery channel by means of a special catheter, similar to those used in coronary angiography but capable of dilating the artery by means of an attached balloon. It may require emergency surgical correction of a damaged artery in 1 to 4 percent of cases. More than one third of patients treated with balloon angioplasty will eventually have recurrence of the obstruction in the treated artery.

c. A number of other procedures are also based on heart catheterization techniques. These include preventing restricture after balloon angioplasty by means of a tube placed within the artery (coronary "stenting") and removing the blockage in the coronary artery from within the artery by means of a laser or a miniature rotating knife (atherectomy).

3. Anesthesia: General

4. Technique: The first step is to remove a short length of either a vein from the patient's leg or an artery from the back of the breast bone. Next, after the heart has been placed at rest by means of the heart-lung machine, one end of that vessel is connected to the patient's aorta (the main artery leading from the heart) and, in the case of vein grafts, the other end is connected to the affected coronary artery, downstream from the area of obstruction, thus bypassing the site of the blockage and restoring adequate blood flow to the heart muscle. Two or more bypass grafts are done in order to bypass all obstructed vessels. Single-artery obstructions are usually handled by balloon angioplasty.

5. Risks:

a. The overall 30-day operative mortality rate for coronary artery bypass grafting should be less than 3 percent in the hospital you have chosen, or you should consider going elsewhere. Several states publish mortality rates for coronary bypass that are specific for individual surgeons and hospitals. If in doubt, ask your surgeon.

b. The risk of heart attack occurring during and after the procedure is about 2 to 4 percent.

c. Complications, such as wound infection, postoperative bleeding, and clotting of the grafts, occur in less than 5 percent of cases.

6. What to Expect:

a. On average, patients stay one or two days in the coronary care unit and are discharged from the hospital in five to seven days. Patients are given anticoagulant drugs such as aspirin, warfarin (Coumadin), or dipyridamole (Persantine), and can usually return to work after two or three months.

b. From 90 to 95 percent of patients benefit from the procedure—that is, their symptoms of chest pain and shortness of breath are improved and they are able to resume a normal lifestyle.

c. Since surgery does not cure coronary-artery disease, symptoms may recur in as many as 40 percent of patients with the passage of time.

Pacemaker Implantation

1. Purpose of the Procedure: To restore the heart's ability to control the rate of its muscular contractions,

primarily to correct bradycardia (abnormally slow heart rate) or pauses of the heartbeat.

2. Nonsurgical Alternatives: Many drugs are available to treat arrhythmias (heart-rhythm disturbances) and should usually be tried first.

3. Anesthesia:

a. Local with sedation for most procedures.

b. General, if heart must be exposed.

4. Technique: Pacemakers are composed of two basic parts, a pulse generator and a pacing wire. The battery-powered pulse generator supplies the heart muscle with regular electrical stimulation through the pacing wire, a special catheter that connects the generator with the heart. Heart pacing can either be temporary (when the condition is transient, as after a heart attack), or permanent (when the abnormal rhythm is recurrent or persistent). Temporary pacing wires are usually placed into the right side of the heart through a neck vein. Permanent pacers require the creation of a small pocket under the skin of the chest wall into which the pulse generator is permanently placed. The pacing wire is usually placed in the heart muscle through a vein in the neck.

5. Risks:

a. The 5 percent possibility of postoperative infection is guarded against by antibiotics.

b. Still less likely is the possibility that the pacing wire will become dislodged or that the pulse generator will fail.

c. Since strong microwave radiation can decrease the electric signal to the heart, patients are advised to avoid exposure to such radiation.

6. What to Expect:

a. The pacemaker can be noticed as a small lump under the skin, but it requires no special attention.

b. Hospital stay is usually one to two days, with return to full activity by one month. (Rough contact sports should be avoided.)

c. Setting the pacemaker to give the optimum signal to the heart (programming it with a device like a TV remote) can take up to three months of office visits.

d. Pacemaker batteries require changing at intervals as long as ten years.

Blood Vessel Surgery

1. Purpose of the Procedures:

a. Endarterectomy: to prevent ulceration or amputation of an arm or leg by restoring the blood supply to the affected limb. Carotid endarterectomy reduces the risk of stroke due to a lack of blood supply to the brain because of blocked arteries.

b. Aneurysmectomy: to prevent the potentially fatal rupture of an aneurysm (a weakening and enlargement of a blood vessel).

c. Arteriorrhaphy: to repair injuries to major blood vessels.

d. Femoropopliteal bypass: To relieve exercise-induced calf, thigh, or buttock pain due to partial arterial obstruction.

e. Arteriovenous fistula: To provide access for dialysis (blood filtering) in patients with kidney failure.

2. Nonsurgical Alternatives:

a. Progressive exercise programs.

b. Aggressive risk-factor management, including smoking cessation, diabetic control, hypertension control, and cholesterol and lipid (fat) control.
c. Surgical support stockings.
d. Local wound care.
e. With the exception of aspirin for carotid-artery disease, medications are rarely effective for symptomatic vascular disease.

3. Anesthesia: General, spinal, epidural, or local

4. Techniques:

a. In carotid endarterectomy: the surgeon removes the diseased plaque or obstruction from within the artery.
b. In aneurysmectomy: the surgeon removes the weakened and dilated artery and replaces it with a tube made of synthetic materials.
c. In aortofemoral bypass: the surgeon places a bypass graft (either a natural vein or a synthetic one) to carry blood around the blocked aorta in the abdomen to an artery in the groin.
d. In femoropopliteal bypass: the surgeon places the graft so as to carry blood from the groin to the knee.
e. In arteriovenous fistula: the surgeon places an artificial tube under the skin, usually of the arm, to make a direct connection between an artery and a vein so as to provide easy access for dialysis.

5. Risks:

a. Operative mortality depends on the overall medical condition of the patient and the location of the vessel being operated on. The more medical problems the patient has, the higher the risk of death. All other factors being equal, age plays a minor role. In general, abdominal procedures carry higher risk to life than operations on the extremities.

b. Hemorrhage occurs in less than 1 percent of cases.
c. The risk of infection is from 0.5 to 3 percent.
d. The most significant complication of vascular surgery is thrombosis, a blood clot within the operated vessel, cutting off the flow of blood beyond the clot. It occurs in 1 to 5 percent of cases and requires emergency reoperation. Thrombosis occurring long after the initial surgery may also be corrected with repeat surgery, but failure to reoperate does not necessarily result in the need to amputate.
e. With carotid surgery there is a 1 to 4 percent risk of stroke. With all other vascular procedures the risk is less than 1 percent.

6. What to Expect:
a. Hospital stays and ultimate recovery vary: for bypass surgery or aneurysm repair, 7 to 10 days in hospital, back to work in three to four weeks; for carotid endarterectomy, two to four days in hospital, back to work in one to two weeks; arteriovenous fistula and venous surgery are ambulatory procedures—in and out of the hospital on the same day; and arteriovenous grafts are completed with an overnight hospital stay.
b. Long-term outlooks also vary. For example, after successful repair of aneurysms, patients have a normal life expectancy. From 60 to 90 percent of patients having endarterectomy succeed in avoiding amputation. Stroke is prevented in 97 percent of patients treated for carotid disease.

MUSCULOSKELETAL PROCEDURES

Arthroscopy (Examination of the inside of a joint)

1. Purpose of the Procedure: To diagnose or treat a disease or injury of a joint—most commonly the knee or shoulder.

2. Nonsurgical Alternatives: Routine diagnostic procedures, such as physical examination and X rays, should always be obtained before arthroscopy is considered.

3. Anesthesia: General anesthesia, although spinal, epidural, and regional nerve blocks may also be used.

4. Technique: The arthroscope—consisting of a tube, an optical system of magnifying lenses, and a fiberoptic light source—is inserted through a very small incision. The surgeon can view the interior of the joint either directly through the instrument or on a video screen. Through another small incision, narrow instruments can be inserted to allow the surgeon to take a biopsy sample, remove loose bits of cartilage, or repair minor tears and other abnormalities. Major joint repairs usually cannot be done through the arthroscope; they require open surgery.

5. Risk: Infection occurs in fewer than 0.5 percent of cases. Antibiotics are frequently given prior to the procedure.

6. What to Expect:

a. Surgeons now perform diagnostic arthroscopy as an outpatient procedure.

b. Recovery from diagnostic arthroscopy is rapid. Some swelling of the joint is expected but disappears within a few days.

c. If major open surgery has been performed, the joint may require immobilization and physical therapy. Hospital stays of 5 to 12 days are usually required.

Open Reduction of Fractures

1. Purpose of the Procedure: To repair complicated bone injuries, especially if there is displacement of bone

fragments and damage to surrounding tissues—most commonly used for fractures of the hip, ankle, and elbow.

2. Nonsurgical Alternatives:

a. Impacted fractures (those in which the bone edges are driven into one another) or fractures that can be adequately realigned by closed methods can often be managed with external support such as casts or splints and restriction of activity.

b. Techniques for uncomplicated fractures can be applied to complicated fractures if the patient's general medical condition precludes surgery. An example would be bed rest and traction for a femoral (thigh bone) fracture rather than surgical repair. Results from nonsurgical approaches to hip and ankle fractures are often disappointing.

3. Anesthesia: General, spinal, or regional

4. Techniques: A variety of metal plates, nails, screws, and rods can be placed into the involved bones to stabilize the fracture site. Such procedures are called "internal fixation." Occasionally, bone grafts, and even artificial materials, may be used to replace bone that has been lost at the fracture site. Some form of external fixation, such as casts, pins, or other devices, is often used after open reduction to provide additional support until healing is complete.

5. Risks:

a. Infection, the chief risk, prevents healing and leads to long-term complications such as nonunion, bone shortening, and chronic pain in 1 percent of cases.

b. Diseases that accompany prolonged bed rest, such as pneumonia and blood clots to the lungs, can occur in as many as 5 to 15 percent of elderly patients.

6. What to Expect:

a. For internal fixation of a fractured hip, you can expect to spend 7 to 10 days in the hospital after surgery, followed by the use of crutches and a walker for four to six weeks. Prolonged sitting is avoided initially, but sedentary work can be resumed in one to two months. Full, unrestricted activity often requires 6 to 12 months.

b. For internal fixation of a fractured ankle, the average hospital stay is two to five days. Patients go home in a cast, which remains in place for four to six weeks. Sedentary work can be resumed in one month when swelling has decreased, and full activity is permitted after three months.

c. Intermittent or low-grade residual pain occurs in 5 percent of cases.

Laminectomy and Spine Fusion

1. Purpose of the Procedure:

a. To relieve pressure on one or more spinal nerves and stabilize the spine to prevent further nerve injury.

b. To relieve symptoms that may include pain, numbness, or weakness of the arm or leg, muscle wasting, or loss of bowel or bladder control.

2. Nonsurgical Alternatives: A conservative approach consists of rest, heat, pain medication, and traction.

3. Anesthesia: General

4. Technique: Surgical approaches vary with the cause of spinal-nerve compression. Injury-induced ruptures of the intervertebral disks, the shock-absorbing tissue cushions between the back bones (often called "herniated disks"), are treated by removal of a portion of the back

bone (laminectomy) to gain access to the displaced disk substance and the removal of it (diskectomy).

When spinal nerves have been compressed by spinal stenosis (excess bone formation in the spine due to arthritis), openings for the nerves to pass between the bones can be enlarged (foraminotomy). Two or more vertebrae can be permanently joined (fused) by means of bone grafts or metal rods. Combinations of laminectomy, foraminotomy, and spinal fusion are often used.

5. Risk: A 10 percent risk of permanent nerve injury makes it especially important to try conservative treatment before even contemplating surgery.

6. What to Expect:

a. For laminectomy: the usual hospital stay is one to three days. Patients can return to light work in two weeks. Physical therapy is often necessary for a period of six weeks to two months.

b. For spinal fusion and foraminotomy: hospital stays are usually a week to 10 days; return to work and duration of physical therapy are highly variable.

c. Although spinal surgery is often successful in reducing nerve-compression symptoms, in some patients pain persists at a lower level of intensity. Other initially successful patients may experience a recurrence of pain with the passage of time.

Arthroplasty (Joint replacement)

1. Purpose of the Procedure:

a. To relieve pain and restore mobility in cases of severe degenerative joint disease (osteoarthritis) limited to a specific joint or pair of joints.

b. Also indicated in some patients with systemic arthritis, such as rheumatoid arthritis, when replacement of a specific joint or joints is necessary.

2. Nonsurgical Alternatives: Conservative measures such as heat, rest, pain medications, weight loss, and the use of walkers, canes, or crutches are usually tried and proven unsuccessful before surgery is considered.

3. Anesthesia: General or spinal

4. Technique: Degenerative joint disease is a disease of the "shock absorber" of the joint (the cartilage that covers the end of the bone). The goal of surgery is to create new surfaces where the bones meet each other. This can be accomplished in one of two ways: by resurfacing one side of the joint, or by replacing the entire joint with a metal or plastic implant. For patients with limited disease, less extreme procedures include realigning the joint by removing a wedge of bone (osteotomy). Totally fusing the joint (arthrodesis) is now infrequently done because, although weight bearing is maintained, joint movement is lost.

5. Risk: In 1 to 2 percent of cases, infection may necessitate removal of the implants. Total joint components may loosen with time in 10 to 20 percent of cases and may require replacement.

6. What to Expect:

a. For arthroplasty of the hip or knee, patients usually stay in the hospital from 5 to 10 days. They begin walking with crutches or a walker and require intensive physiotherapy for two to four months. They usually return to work in three or four months. Replacement of finger joints also requires extensive physiotherapy, but usually allows an earlier return to work.

b. All artificial joints fail eventually and, depending on the age of the patient, may require replacement. With certain finger joints, the time to failure can be as short as several months. Hip and knee arthroplasties usually last for many years. The need for replacement is usually heralded by a return of pain.

c. The danger of infection continues long after the wound has healed, so patients are often advised to treat any future infections with a full course of antibiotics to prevent infection of the implant.

GYNECOLOGICAL SURGERY

Hysterectomy (Removal of the uterus)

1. Purpose of the Procedure:

a. To treat tumors or abnormal growths, such as cancer, endometriosis (the spread of tissue that lines the uterus to other parts of the abdominal cavity), or fibroids (benign smooth-muscle tumors).

b. To remove a ruptured uterus or one that has been severely damaged during vaginal delivery after cesarean.

c. To remove a prolapsed uterus, one that has fallen from its normal position because of tearing or weakening of the supporting muscles and ligaments during childbirth.

d. To treat excessive menstrual bleeding or pain.

2. Nonsurgical Alternatives:

a. For asymptomatic fibroids: watchful waiting.

b. For endometriosis: hormonal and steroidal drugs.

c. For prolapse: pelvic-muscle exercises, or the insertion of a pessary (a metal, plastic, or rubber ring-shaped supporting device that fits around the cervix).
d. For heavy bleeding and excessive pain: anti-inflammatory drugs, hormones, endometrial ablation (excision), dilation and curettage.

3. Anesthesia: General or regional

4. Techniques: Hysterectomy can be performed through an abdominal incision or by an approach through the vagina. In general, abdominal hysterectomy is reserved for patients with a greatly enlarged uterus and those with suspected cancer.
a. Subtotal hysterectomy (removal of the body of the uterus but leaving the cervix) is increasingly common today, especially in patients with fibroids. Total hysterectomy is the complete removal of the uterus. When malignant disease is present, hysterectomy is combined with removal of both Fallopian tubes and ovaries (hysterectomy with bilateral salpingo-oophorectomy). Radical hysterectomy refers to removal of the uterus, both tubes and ovaries, and the surrounding soft tissues and lymphatics for more advanced cancers. All of those procedures are done through an incision in the lower abdomen.
b. Since vaginal hysterectomy requires shorter hospital stays and results in speedier recovery, it is chosen whenever possible. With this procedure, all incisions are placed within the vagina, and the uterus is removed through the vagina.
c. Laparoscopic removal of uterine tumors is becoming increasingly common.

5. Risks:
a. Overall mortality risk is 0.1 percent but is slightly higher for cases involving pregnancy or cancer.

b. Complications, such as infection (1 to 5 percent), hemorrhage (1 percent), pulmonary embolism (0.5 to 1 percent), and operative injury to adjacent organs are rare.

6. What to Expect:

a. Hospital stays for hysterectomy range from three to six days, with resumption of normal activity in as little as two to three weeks. Intercourse may be resumed after four to six weeks.

b. When both ovaries have been removed along with the uterus, patients experience abrupt onset of menopausal symptoms. Estrogen replacement is then often recommended to relieve hot flashes. A long-range benefit of that treatment is the prevention of osteoporosis (weakening of the bones) and possibly of coronary heart disease.

c. Chronic fatigue, depression, and loss or reduction of libido occur in 10 to 20 percent of patients. Alternatively, many women respond to the relief of symptoms, cessation of abnormal vaginal bleeding, or removal of the risk of future pregnancy by a marked improvement in emotional outlook.

d. With vaginal hysterectomy, complications are fewer, there is less pain, and recovery is somewhat faster.

Salpingo-Oophorectomy (Removal of ovary and Fallopian tube)

1. Purpose of the Procedure:

a. To remove tumors of the ovary.

b. To terminate an ectopic pregnancy (removal of tube only).

c. To treat chronic infection of the tube and ovary.

d. To eliminate hormones in selected breast-cancer patients.

e. To prevent ovarian cancer in patients with a strong family history of that disease.

2. Nonsurgical Alternatives:

a. For some women under 30 years of age: watchful waiting, since 90 percent of their ovarian tumors are benign. (At age 50, half of ovarian growths are malignant.)
b. For ectopic pregnancy: the drug methotrexate is now being used. If the tube ruptures, it is usually a life-threatening emergency and there is no nonsurgical alternative.
c. For infection: a course of antibiotics should be tried.

3. Anesthesia: General

4. Technique: Salpingo-oophorectomy can be done as a unilateral procedure, for certain benign tumors or ectopic pregnancy, or bilaterally, for breast cancer and (with hysterectomy) for ovarian malignancy. An incision is made in the abdomen allowing the surgeon to pick up and excise the tube and ovary. Laparoscopic techniques are being increasingly used.

5. Risk: Mortality risk is less than 0.1 percent.

6. What to Expect:

a. Hospital stays vary from two to six days. With laparoscopic procedures, patients stay only a day or two.
b. Long-term, even lifetime estrogen replacement is usually advised if both ovaries have been removed.

Tubal Ligation (Female sterilization)

1. Purpose of the Procedure: To prevent future pregnancy.

2. Nonsurgical Alternatives: Various forms of contraception, such as birth-control pills, condoms, cervical cap, diaphragm, hormone injections or implants, IUDs, spermicides, sponge, and vasectomy (male sterilization).

3. Anesthesia: General or regional

4. Technique: Most tubal ligations are now being done laparoscopically. The laparoscope is inserted through the abdominal wall near the navel. Each Fallopian tube is picked up by instruments manipulated through the laparoscope, and either clamped shut with clips or sealed shut with an electric current or, less commonly, a laser; some surgeons prefer to remove a section of each tube and then occlude the remaining ends.

5. Risks:

a. Mortality is exceedingly rare.

b. Surgical accidents, such as bowel perforation, have been reported but seldom occur.

6. What to Expect:

a. Tubal ligation is usually done as an outpatient procedure, and work can be resumed in two to three days.

b. Sterilization is complete when a section of each tube has been removed or when both tubes have been effectively blocked. Clipping, tying, or burning tubes may result in a less than 1 percent risk of continued fertility.

c. Tuboplasty (surgery to reverse tubal ligation) can be attempted, with only a 20 to 40 percent chance of success, depending on the method used in the sterilization procedure. Reversal is most difficult if sections of the tube have been removed. For practical purposes, tubal ligation should not be considered if any possibility exists that pregnancy might be desired in the future.

Dilation and Curettage (Scraping the lining of the uterus)

1. Purpose of the Procedure:

a. To examine and diagnose abnormalities in the lining of the uterus manifested by abnormal or irregular bleeding.

b. To remove polyps or tumors from the uterus.

c. To remove any fetal or placental material that remains after a miscarriage.

d. To control excessive menstrual bleeding.

2. Nonsurgical Alternatives: For excessive menstrual bleeding, hormones.

3. Technique: The vagina is widened with a speculum, and through it, the cervix (the mouth of the uterus) is gradually enlarged with dilators until the opening is large enough to admit a scraping instrument. The lining of the uterus (endometrium) is removed with repeated passages of the instrument.

4. Anesthesia: General, regional, or local

5. Risks:

a. Perforation of the uterus is a rare complication, which may require additional surgery.

b. The possibility of infection may be guarded against by antibiotics.

6. What to Expect:

a. These are outpatient procedures. Most normal activity can usually be resumed within 24 hours, but sexual intercourse should be delayed for five or six days.

b. Postoperative bleeding or discharge is rare.

Repair of Cystocele, Rectocele, Enterocele, Uterine Prolapse

1. Purpose of the Procedure:

a. To correct protrusions into the vagina of the bladder (cystocele), the rectum (rectocele), the small intestine (enterocele), or the uterus, caused by a weakening of the supporting ligaments and muscles, resulting from pregnancy and childbirth.

b. To relieve symptoms caused by these hernias, such as stress incontinence (involuntary loss of urine with coughing, sneezing, or laughing), difficulty in having bowel movements (except by pushing the vagina backward against the rectum), constipation, and a constant sensation of pressure in the pelvis.

2. Nonsurgical Treatment: Conservative management, such as the use of a pessary, may provide relief.

3. Anesthesia: General or regional

4. Techniques: A vaginal approach is preferred, since it permits the surgeon to repair any associated problems. These procedures are often combined with a vaginal hysterectomy. To correct cystocele or rectocele (protrusion of the bladder or rectum), the surgeon strengthens the vaginal wall by closing defects in the dense surrounding tissues. To repair enterocele (hernia of the small intestine), the surgeon reconstructs the pelvic floor. In cases of severe uterine prolapse, vaginal hysterectomy is combined with repair of the pelvic floor.

5. Risk: Mortality risk is extremely low—less than 1 percent.

6. What to Expect:

a. Hospital stays range from three to seven days, depending on what is repaired. Patients can return to work in four to six weeks.

b. Sexual intercourse may be resumed four to six weeks after surgery.

c. Approximately 20 percent of patients will experience recurrence of symptoms with time.

GENITOURINARY PROCEDURES

Cystoscopy (Internal examination of the bladder)

1. Purpose of the Procedure:

a. To inspect the inner surface of the urethra, bladder, and prostate in order to diagnose disorders such as infections, injuries, polyps, stones, and tumors.

b. To remove or crush small tumors, stones, or polyps.

c. To remove a sample of tissue for microscopic examination (biopsy).

2. Nonsurgical Alternatives: Other diagnostic procedures, including urinalysis, blood tests, X-ray studies, computerized tomography (CT scanning), and ultrasound, should ordinarily precede cystoscopy.

3. Anesthesia: General, regional, or local with sedation

4. Technique: The cystoscope (a rigid or flexible tube with a telescopic viewing lens that transmits light) is inserted through the urethra into the bladder. After filling the bladder with sterile water, the urologist is able to inspect the entire inner surface. Biopsies of the lining of the

bladder are taken as necessary, and the urethra can be inspected as the cystoscope is removed.

5. Risks:

a. Bladder irritation and infection occasionally result.

b. Perforation of the bladder and hemorrhage are rare complications.

6. What to Expect:

a. Cystoscopy is usually an outpatient procedure, and normal activities can be resumed in 24 hours.

b. Antibiotics are usually prescribed.

c. Some mild burning sensation with urination is common but lasts only a day or two.

Prostatectomy (Removal of the prostate gland)

1. Purpose of the Procedure:

a. To relieve the symptoms of benign prostatic hypertrophy (BPH, a noncancerous enlargement of the prostate gland). Symptoms include frequency of urination, urinary retention, and poor urinary flow, all caused by pressure on the neck of the bladder by the enlarged prostate gland.

b. To treat prostate cancer limited to the gland itself.

2. Nonsurgical Alternatives:

a. For BPH, watchful waiting until the inability to completely empty the bladder results in significant changes in lifestyle or the risk of serious bladder and kidney problems.

b. For BPH, drug therapy with alpha-blockers, finasteride (Proscar), or both may reduce the size of the gland and reduce symptoms. If successful, the drugs must be taken indefinitely.

c. For BPH, some new nonsurgical approaches are becoming available. They include microwave treatment, balloon dilation, and inserting a stent. Be warned, however: Some of these procedures are used only on men with a prostate of a certain size and shape; some are considered experimental and may not be covered by health insurers; most do not have a long-term track record, as does the standard surgery; and many can be done only at certain medical centers with the appropriate equipment.

d. Some studies suggest that men with early prostate cancer, diagnosed while it is still confined to the gland, can do well without surgical treatment. Since prostate cancer is usually a slow-growing tumor, treatment of elderly patients may not be necessary.

e. For localized prostate cancer, radiation can be applied externally over a period of six weeks, or internally by means of radioactive seeds implanted into the prostate in an individually prescribed pattern.

f. Decreasing the level of the male hormone testosterone slows the growth of prostate cancer and causes the tumor to shrink. This can be accomplished by the surgical removal of the testicles, by monthly injections of a synthetic hormone that blocks the production of testosterone by the testes, and by tablets that block the effects of testosterone in the body.

3. Anesthesia: General or regional

4. Techniques:

a. The most common surgical approach to BPH is a procedure called "transurethral resection of the prostate" (TURP). The surgeon passes a flexible instrument called a "resectoscope" into the penis and up into the urethra. A viewing system shows the narrowed portions of the urethra from the inside; the surgeon cuts the prostatic tissue into strips with an electric current or coagulates it with a laser beam to widen the constricted passage. (As a precaution, tissue is checked for cancer after it is removed.) In time the shell of prostate remaining after surgery grows a new section.

b. Larger benign lesions of the prostate can be removed through an incision made between the pubic bone and the navel. In a suprapubic procedure, the bladder is opened and the obstructive prostate tissue is removed, leaving the prostate shell behind. In a retropubic procedure, access is gained behind the pubic bone directly to the prostate. Again the interior of the prostate is removed, leaving the shell behind. A perineal prostatectomy is performed through an incision made just in front of the anus.

c. Cancers of the prostate that can be removed surgically are often approached by the perineal technique, although many surgeons use the retropubic approach.

5. Risks:

a. Overall mortality rates range from 0.1 percent for TURP, to 1 percent for cancer surgery.

b. Postoperative bleeding is a common complication.

c. Loss of sexual potency occurs in 30 to 40 percent of patients, even with nerve-sparing techniques.

d. Urinary incontinence is common after all forms of prostatectomy but usually improves with time and is only persistent in 1 to 3 percent of cases.

6. What to Expect:

a. Hospital stay about one week. Patients go home with catheter and drainage bag for another two weeks.

b. Since the entire prostate is not removed for BPH (only the portion pressing against the urethra), recurrence of obstruction occurs in 10 percent of patients.

c. Retrograde ejaculation of semen back into the bladder

rather than out of the urethra is common after TURP and results in sterility. The sexual response is otherwise intact.

d. Lifelong follow-up for prostate cancer is required.

SKIN SURGERY

Skin Biopsy

1. Purpose of the Procedure:

a. To diagnose skin diseases.

b. To remove small localized skin lesions.

2. Nonsurgical Alternative: "Chemosurgery" (direct application of cancer-destroying agents to small superficial cancers).

3. Techniques:

a. For small lesions: excisional biopsy removes the entire skin lesion.

b. For large lesions, which would leave unsightly scars if removed completely: incisional biopsy removes only a part of the lesion.

4. Anesthesia: Local, with sedation as necessary

5. Risk: Slight risk of infection or bleeding.

6. What to Expect: Depending on the tissue diagnosis, further treatment may be necessary.

Skin Graft

1. Purpose of the Procedure: To replace skin lost from surgery, accidents, extensive burns, large ulcers, and the like.

2. Nonsurgical Alternatives: Artificial skin substitutes, cadaver or donor skin, or even animal skin, can be used, but only as short-term coverage.

3. Anesthesia: General or regional

4. Techniques:

a. In split-section grafting, extremely thin (less than 1 millimeter) sections of skin are taken from one area of the body, often the front of the thigh, and transferred to the area that needs coverage. The graft is secured over the defect with a pressure dressing and sometimes a few stitches. The skin defect created at the donor site usually heals within two weeks.

b. Full-thickness skin grafts are usually taken in conjunction with underlying muscle and blood vessels ("free flaps"). They can be moved to any part of the body requiring a thicker coverage, where they are reconnected to the local blood vessels.

5. Risks:

a. Sometimes the skin graft will not take, and repeated grafting becomes necessary.

b. Infections can occur at the donor site.

6. What to Expect:

a. Hospital stays range from 6 to 12 days.

b. Oozing of blood from the donor site lasts one or two days.

c. Since the primary purpose of skin grafting is to provide coverage, the cosmetic result may be somewhat disappointing. It's unlikely that the color and texture of the new skin will exactly match the surrounding area.

BREAST SURGERY

Mastectomy (Removal of all or some portion of the breast)

1. Purpose of the Procedure:

a. To diagnose a breast mass by biopsy.

b. To treat breast cancer.

2. Nonsurgical Alternatives:

a. For early detection of breast cancer, mammography—a specialized X-ray study of breast tissue—is the best tool we have. It can detect cancer cells up to two years before a woman or her doctor could feel a small lump. But mammograms are fallible. They miss about 1 of every 10 breast cancers in women over age 50 and about half of cancers in women younger than that.

To keep track of changes between mammograms, all women should examine their own breasts every month. They should also undergo a professional examination at least once a year.

b. For the treatment of breast cancer, radiation or chemotherapy have not given as good results alone as when combined with surgery.

3. Anesthesia: General, or local with sedation

4. Techniques:

a. For diagnostic purposes, a small portion of a breast mass is removed, either through a special hollow needle that draws a few cells out of the lump (fine-needle biopsy) or through a larger needle that takes a small piece out of the lump (tru-cut biopsy), by taking a somewhat larger piece of lump (incisional biopsy), or by removing the entire lump (excisional biopsy).

b. Once a diagnosis of breast cancer has been made, decisions must be made about how extensive the surgery will be—that is, how much breast tissue will be removed. The choice of procedure depends on the size of the tumor, its location in the breast, the type of cancer cells that are involved and their rate of growth, and whether or not the cancer has spread. Surgery is usually followed up with a course of radiation therapy, hormone therapy, or chemotherapy.

- Lumpectomy is the complete excision of a relatively small malignant tumor, along with a substantial amount of normal tissue surrounding it. As much as one quarter of the breast tissue may be removed.
- In a simple mastectomy, the surgeon removes the entire breast. Some lymph nodes may be taken from the armpit to see if any malignant cells are present.
- Modified radical mastectomy consists of removal of the entire breast together with all of the lymph nodes of the armpit, leaving the muscles of the chest wall undisturbed.
- Radical mastectomy consists of removal of the entire breast, all of the lymph nodes in the armpit, and the underlying muscles of the chest wall.

5. Risks: Obviously, the degree of risk increases with the extent of the surgical procedure, ranging from a 1 percent risk of hemorrhage or infection for a biopsy to 2 to 5 percent for radical mastectomy. The mortality rate for modified radical is 1 percent and for radical mastectomy, it's 1 to 2 percent.

6. What to Expect:

a. Biopsies are often performed in a doctor's office or in a hospital's ambulatory surgery department, with no overnight stay. For the other procedures, hospital stays range up to 5 to 10 days for radical mastectomy.

b. As more and more breast tissue and underlying tissues are removed, the need for physical therapy increases. This consists of exercises designed to maintain flexibility and mobility of the shoulder.

c. Following mastectomy, or sometimes before surgery, a patient may decide to have her breast reconstructed—either with an artificial implant or with tissue taken usually from her back or abdomen; this may be done at the same time as the mastectomy or at a later date. Some women decide to wear a prosthesis, a sort of falsie designed to fit inside a bra. And some women opt for neither.

d. Massive swelling of the arm after breast surgery (known as lymphedema) is rarely seen following modern breast-cancer operations, since the older technique that required extensive removal of the lymph nodes (which simultaneously drain both the breast and the arm) has not been shown to increase survival significantly.

e. The optimal therapy for breast cancer remains controversial and individual. In recent years, lumpectomy combined with radiation and chemotherapy has provided survival results as good as those for more destructive surgical procedures. The relative values of radiation, chemotherapy, and new drugs such as tamoxifen, which blocks the effects of the hormone estrogen in the body, are still being established.

f. Lifelong follow-up is required to monitor recurrence, as well as to guard against the development of cancer in the opposite breast.

THORACIC SURGERY

Bronchoscopy (Examination of the air passages)

1. Purpose of the Procedure:

a. To diagnose diseases within the air passages (trachea and bronchi) or lungs.

b. To remove a foreign body, mucus plugs, or blood from the air passages.

c. To control bleeding from the lung.

2. Nonsurgical Alternatives:

a. Noninvasive studies, including X-ray, CT scan, MRI, and pulmonary function tests, should precede diagnostic bronchoscopy.

b. To remove accumulations of secretions, postural drainage and chest percussion may be helpful. Physiotherapy and deep-breathing exercises should also be tried before bronchoscopy is used for this purpose.

3. Anesthesia: General, or local with sedation

4. Technique: Bronchoscopy can be performed, under sedation, with either a rigid or a flexible bronchoscope. Following local anesthesia of the throat to suppress cough and gag reflexes, the bronchoscope is introduced into the air passages (bronchi) through the mouth. Direct visualization of the air passages permits biopsies to be taken if required, or direct treatment can be applied to the bronchi.

5. Risk: The overall risk is quite low but increases when lung function is compromised, since the oxygen-carrying capacity of the blood may be reduced during the procedure.

6. What to Expect: Bronchscopy is usually an outpatient procedure. Afterward, many patients experience a slight sore throat, which quickly resolves.

Pulmonary Resection (Removal of all or part of a lung)

1. Purpose of the Procedure:

a. To prevent the spread of lung cancer to other parts of the body.

b. To remove a nonfunctioning lung or portion of lung that has been destroyed or severely damaged by infections resistant to drug therapy, or by emphysema, hemorrhage, or trauma.

c. To establish a diagnosis of a lesion seen on X ray.

2. Nonsurgical Alternatives: If cancer is suspected, a transcutaneous biopsy can be performed: An X-ray-guided needle is inserted through the skin into the lung so that a sample of tissue can be removed for microscopic analysis.

3. Anesthesia: General

4. Techniques: The lung is approached through an incision into the chest wall, usually below the nipple and extending around to the back, below the shoulder blade. Surgical exposure may necessitate removal of a rib. Varying amounts of lung may be removed, depending on the extent of the disease: total removal of one lung (pneumonectomy), removal of one of the five lung segments (lobectomy), or removal of a smaller portion of lung (segmentectomy). The major air passages are closed off by sutures or staples. Recently, endoscopic surgery (called "thoracoscopic surgery" when used in the chest) has been

successfully employed for lung biopsies and for removal of segments and lobes.

5. Risks:

a. The overall mortality rate for removal of an entire lung is 2 to 5 percent, depending on the overall condition of the patient. The risk is lower when less lung tissue is removed.

b. Major complications such as air leak, hemorrhage, and infection are possible.

6. What to Expect:

a. Hospital stays range from 4 to 10 days, depending on the amount of lung removed. Pneumonectomy usually involves two to three days in an intensive care unit. Drainage tubes placed in the chest at the time of surgery are removed in two to four days if no air leak is present. Work can be resumed in two to four months.

b. If less than one lung has been removed, significant shortness of breath or restrictions on physical activity are rarely seen following recovery.

CENTRAL NERVOUS SYSTEM SURGERY

Craniotomy (Brain surgery)

1. Purpose of the Procedure:

a. To remove tumors.

b. To treat blood vessel abnormalities, such as malformations, rupture, and hemorrhage.

c. To treat injuries to the brain.

2. Nonsurgical Alternatives:

a. To kill tumor cells or halt the spread of disease: radiation and/or chemotherapy are rarely as successful as surgery.

b. To diminish swelling and reduce pressure: corticosteroid drugs.

c. To control seizures: anticonvulsant drugs.

d. For pain: analgesics.

e. Highly concentrated X-ray therapy ("the Gamma Knife") can be used in place of surgery in certain conditions, such as blood vessel malformation (arteriovenous fistulas).

3. Anesthesia: General, or local with sedation

4. Technique: The brain is usually approached by creating a large flap of scalp and skull bone over the area of interest. Since brain tissue has more blood supply than other tissues, meticulous control of bleeding is required. Small lesions within the brain can be handled by stereotactic surgery, in which destructive probes are placed into the brain through small holes drilled in the skull. The probes are guided to the area of abnormality by precise X-ray localization techniques.

5. Risks:

a. Overall mortality rates vary significantly from 1 to 30 percent or more, depending on the type and degree of the underlying condition.

b. Hemorrhage, infection, paralysis, aphasia (loss of the ability to speak) may occur.

6. What to Expect:

a. Hospital stays range from 5 to 10 days. Return to work depends on the diagnosis, but not usually before 3 to 12 weeks.

b. Changes in the ability to control movements of the

body, and to smell, see, hear, speak, and think are possible after craniotomy, depending on the location of the lesion and the amount of brain tissue removed.

c. Headaches are common for the first week but should be rare two to four weeks later.

EYE SURGERY

Cataract Extraction (Removal of the lens)

1. Purpose of the Procedure: To restore sight impaired by clouding of the lens due to normal aging, trauma, diabetes mellitus, or long-term use of corticosteroid drugs (eye drops or oral pills). Cigarette smoking and chronic exposure to high levels of radiation from X rays, microwaves, or even the sun may also play a role in cataract formation.

2. Nonsurgical Alternatives: Once a cataract has formed, a slowly progressive process gradually diminishes vision in the affected eye. Only removal of the lens will restore the patient's vision. The decision to remove a cataract depends on the general health of the patient and how much the decrease in vision due to the cataract interferes with daily activities. To achieve maximum benefit from the procedure, the patient's vision should be worse than 20/60 before surgery. As a less than perfect alternative to surgery, contact lenses or extremely thick eyeglasses may be worn, but vision will still be somewhat impaired.

3. Anesthesia: Local with sedation

4. Technique: After dilating the pupil with eye drops, the surgeon makes incisions in the sclera or cornea (the

coverings of the eye) and another incision in the anterior lens capsule through which the lens can be withdrawn, leaving intact the posterior capsule behind the lens. A synthetic plastic replacement lens is then inserted into the cavity left empty by the removed lens and the incision is closed with very fine sutures.

5. Risks:

a. Retinal tear and detachment, hemorrhage, infection, and displacement of the artificial lens are possible complications.

b. In 30 to 40 percent of cases, the initially clear posterior capsule may become opaque after cataract surgery, requiring a simple outpatient procedure with the laser.

6. What to Expect:

a. Cataract extraction is an outpatient procedure, and discomfort is usually mild. Patients can return to work in two to three weeks. Vigorous exercise, such as jogging, can be resumed after two months.

b. The operated eye is usually patched for 12 to 24 hours, after which the patch is worn only at night for about one month.

c. Corrective lenses are required in almost all cases for optimal vision.

d. Full recovery of vision often takes weeks, but it can be expected in 90 to 95 percent of cases.

13

QUALITY CONTROL

Quality-control measures are applied to many areas of health care. Physicians, medical-equipment companies, drug manufacturers, hospitals, and many other players in the health-care field are monitored—with varying degrees of stringency—by local, state, and federal agencies. Increasingly, third-party payers such as insurance companies and employers also participate in quality control as part of their efforts to contain costs.

Control of the quality of surgeons and surgical care is a cooperative effort of educators, professionals, and government officials. Various agencies and organizations regulate and standardize the content of medical education in medical schools, during residency training, and in continuing medical education programs. How well an individual surgeon absorbs these educational offerings and applies them to the care of patients in the actual practice of medicine or surgery is also monitored and to some extent even controlled.

EDUCATION—AN ONGOING PROCESS

Quality control begins at the earliest stages of a surgical career. Applicants are screened and tested as each medical school strives to select only those capable of mastering the complexities of its curriculum. Once admitted to medical school, students are continuously observed and tested in an effort to weed out unqualified candidates. The quality of the medical school itself and its curriculum is subject to review by a national regulatory body, the Liaison Committee for Medical Education (LCME), which sets national standards that must be met by all the schools.

The quality of residency training programs is supervised by the Accreditation Council for Graduate Medical Education (ACGME). This broad-based organization has representatives from all branches of organized medicine and maintains 25 residency review committees (RRCs) that act as field representatives for the parent organization. They review the educational and practical components of the training programs by making comprehensive on-site observations at intervals of three to five years. The RRCs report to the Accreditation Council, which in turn approves or denies accreditation.

As a result of the RRC reports, training programs that don't conform to the ACGME quality guidelines can lose accreditation entirely or be placed on probation. Those denied accreditation must discontinue their residency programs until all deficiencies are corrected. The ACGME also conducts studies aimed at improving postgraduate medical education and reviews and approves proposals for new training programs.

Surgical residents who fail to meet the intellectual, technical, or personal standards of their training institution are dropped from the program. Those who are rejected by one training program are free to try to find a position in another institution, but this is becoming increasingly more difficult for surgical residents, as demand for training positions remains high. Often the rejected trainee will decide to choose another specialty rather than try to find a place to continue in surgery.

Candidates successfully completing a surgical residency must then apply to one of the specialty boards. The American Board of Medical Specialties (ABMS), originally established in 1933 and now comprising 29 member boards from all branches of medicine, is responsible for setting and maintaining the standards for board certification of surgeons and physicians in all the specialties. It also establishes procedures designed to ensure continued competence after initial certification, such as time-limited certification and mandatory recertification.

Postgraduate Education

Like many professions, medicine is struggling valiantly to overcome the effects of the information explosion. The good news is that an overwhelming volume of new medical information is being generated. The bad news is that it has become impossible for any individual to remain current in all aspects of medicine. Information accumulates and changes with increasing speed. It is estimated that the entire database of medical information changes every six years. This means that surgeons who fail to continue their medical education after graduation will become obsolete in less time than it took for them to become surgeons. Continuing medical education (CME) is therefore a necessity if surgical competence is to be maintained.

The Council of Medical Specialty Societies (CMSS) was organized in 1965 to improve the quality of medical care in the United States and foster excellence in the continuing postgraduate education of physicians. Twenty-four societies, representing each of the specialty disciplines in medicine, belong to the Council.

Because of the importance of continuing medical education, another organization with an even wider range of membership has come into being. The Accreditation Council for Continuing Medical Education (ACCME) is sponsored by the American Board of Medical Specialties, the American Hospital Association, the American Medical Association, the Association of American Medical Colleges, the Council of Medical Specialty Societies, and the Federation of State Medical Boards of the United States. ACCME fosters, evaluates, accredits, and standardizes programs in continuing medical education at local, state, and national levels.

There are many ways for a physician to continue his or her medical education and keep current after completing the years of formal training. Most physicians subscribe to at least one monthly periodical, a professional journal with reports of recent scientific research and clinical studies related to diagnosis and treatment in their field of primary interest. Most hospitals and medical societies have a medical library that receives many such journals to supplement its collection of medical books and monographs. Unsolicited medical information, published by various private-interest entities, arrives daily in doctors' offices all over the country. There are medical radio programs, videotapes, audiotapes, electronic databases, and television programs—of varying objectivity and reliability, of course, since many are sponsored by commercial interests.

Hospitals and medical societies sponsor lectures and teaching days, grand rounds in which clinical cases are reviewed, and other programs. Medical schools offer special programs in connection with annual reunions and other alumni functions. More than 300 national medical meetings, sanctioned by the ACGME for continuing medical education, are held each year. One of the most important of such meetings for surgeons is the Clinical Congress of the American College of Surgeons, which is open to all surgeons, whether Fellows of the American College or not. In short, every conceivable form and type of continuing medical education is available to any physician wishing to invest the time in self-education.

Although organized medicine provides this elaborate framework for continuing medical education, the programs must succeed or fail one physician at a time. With few exceptions, participation in these programs is entirely voluntary. The AMA has not made continuing medical education mandatory, although it does offer Physician's Recognition Awards for voluntary participation in CME programs. Similarly, the American College of Surgeons offers the Surgical Self-Assessment Program (SSAP), a voluntary course in continuing surgical education.

Only 22 states have passed legislation requiring proof of a physician's participation in CME programs for renewal of the license to practice medicine. The amount of CME time required to retain those licenses ranges from 25 to 100 hours a year, for an average of 50 hours. Many would regard that amount of time as a minimum requirement.

Only seven specialty boards—emergency medicine, family practice, general surgery, obstetrics and gynecology, orthopedics, thoracic surgery, and urology—have begun to require recertification examinations at specified intervals. The examinations stress current methods of diagnosis and treatment. Individuals who either fail the recertification examination or neglect to take it lose their board certification. Eight additional boards have plans for mandatory recertification.

Recertification has been mandatory in general surgery since 1976. For many other specialties, compliance with CME programs and opportunities is voluntary, but mandatory CME and specialty board recertification is gaining support.

IMPAIRMENT AND INCOMPETENCE

Like people everywhere, physicians can suffer from physical limitations, mental illness, substance abuse, or other disabilities. Their skills may become obsolete, they may become negligent, or they may be downright incompetent. In an acute-care specialty such as surgery, such disabilities become magnified. Although organized medicine has established guidelines for surveillance of its members and enforcement of its ethical principles, some disabilities are more difficult than others to detect. Patient care may be severely compromised by any of these mental or physical disabilities, yet the affected physicians may continue to escape detection.

Drug and Alcohol Addiction

The vast majority of surgeons, like most people, manage the stresses and strains of their professional and private lives appropriately. Some, however, do not. Studies show that as many as 82,500—10 to 15 percent of the nation's 550,000 physicians—may suffer from substance abuse or mental illness. Alcoholism is the leading form of physician impairment, occurring twice as frequently as either drug addiction or mental illness. Identification of impaired physicians before any harm comes to their patients has become a focus of increasing regional and national effort.

Since denial is a principal defense in individuals with substance addiction, it's as rare for physicians to seek help as it is for nonphysicians. Most often, substance-impaired physicians are reported to enforcement agencies by hospital administrators, pharmacists, family members, and colleagues. Medical and surgical colleagues are often in the best position to recognize substance abuse and mental illness among their coworkers. Although the AMA has declared it unethical for a physician to fail to "take cognizance of a colleague's inability to practice medicine adequately by reason of physical or mental illness, including alcoholism or drug dependence," there has always been a code of silence among physicians. But fraternalism at the expense of the public can no longer be tolerated. To restore and maintain the public's confidence in the medical profession, there must be a more visible commitment of the profession to police itself.

Physical and Mental Impairment

Impaired physical performance has received scant attention from the medical profession or its regulatory agencies.

It's well known that eye-hand coordination declines with advancing age, yet surgeons have a hard time quitting. All too often, they hang on at the end of a distinguished career denying—to themselves most of all—that they may be putting their patients at significant risk.

Many hospitals have established mandatory retirement for surgeons, typically at age 65. While some surgeons can operate effectively beyond that age and may therefore ask that an exception be made in their case, others cannot. The process of granting individual exceptions invites charges of discrimination and litigation, so hospitals often maintain a strict retirement policy. In general, mandatory retirement is in the best interests of the public.

Deterioration of a surgeon's skills because of disease or injury is rarely discussed. Often the individual surgeon is left to decide for himself or herself whether the condition is temporary, and how much operative technique has been affected. Organized medicine has not faced up to this issue. Several states include issues of physician impairment in so-called sick-doctor statutes. Physicians who are unable to practice with reasonable skill and safety by reason of illness, injury, addiction, mental disorders, old age, or loss of motor skills are required to undergo an impartial medical examination. Of course, probable cause to submit to this examination must be shown. Failure to pass the medical examination can lead to modifications in hospital or operative privileges, or even suspension or revocation of the license to practice.

Incompetence: The Real Danger

Incompetence is the most difficult disability to detect. It's often easier to recognize and rehabilitate an impaired physician than it is to identify and reeducate an incompetent one. The dictionary definition of incompetence is "an inability to perform at an expected level." But how do you establish that? Who is to be the judge? No two surgeons have identical views. One surgeon's example of incompetence may be another surgeon's treatment of choice. Charges of incompetence are extremely difficult to establish in the absence of gross negligence. Furthermore, competence is not an absolute. A surgeon may be quite competent in some areas and completely adrift in others. Incompetence is often a judgment call rather than a verifiable fact.

Ideally, judgments that result in restrictions of surgical practice are best made by a surgeon's peers. From a practical standpoint, however, this rarely happens. Surgeons may harbor low opinions of some of their colleagues, but most often they hesitate to file a formal complaint. Charging a colleague with incompetence offers few rewards to the accusing surgeon. Furthermore, allegations of incompetence by one surgeon against another could be regarded as being motivated by self-interest. Any attorney would be quick to point out a possible conflict of interest on the part of one surgeon testifying against another.

To protect individuals from frivolous or malicious accusations, it's important that all censoring actions for incompetence proceed carefully and with due process. But even when physicians and hospitals act with the purest motives of safeguarding the welfare of patients, when they seek to restrict the practice of an incompetent surgeon, the threat of a countersuit always exists.

Many hospitals prefer to permit an incompetent surgeon to resign from the staff rather than undertake the lengthy and expensive course of censorship or restriction of privileges by due process. Unfortunately, that approach may only move the problem along to the next hospital, in which the incompetent surgeon continues the substandard practices and exposes the public to continued risk. Clearly, it's easier to prevent licensure of the incompetent physician than it is to revoke the license to practice once it has been granted. State licensing agencies are aware of this fact and make considerable efforts to identify incompetence before a physician is licensed.

But what of the physician who was competent at the time of licensure but has become incompetent through indifference or neglect? Mandatory programs for measuring and monitoring the competence of physicians and surgeons would go a long way toward restoring public confidence in the medical profession. But even without such programs, unknown to the public, censure actions, restrictions of surgical privileges, and limitation or revocation of the license to practice medicine occur throughout the country on a daily basis. While no one suggests that the quality-control functions are foolproof or uniformly effective, organized medicine has come a long way from the old days of fraternal neglect. There are safeguards, and there are agencies to enforce them.

SAFEGUARDS AND SECURITY

The local hospital is the public's first line of defense against impaired or incompetent surgeons. The principle is simple: No one knows surgeons better than their peers, the colleagues with whom they work every day. But higher levels of authority also come into play in the process of reviewing and maintaining high-quality surgical performance.

The Local Hospital

To be granted operating privileges in any hospital, a surgeon must first satisfy the hospital's Credentials Committee and Chief of Surgery of the quality of his or her training. Each candidate must present a list of all the operations he or she wishes to perform. Both hospital and surgical privileges are reviewed every two to three years and appropriate changes are made.

Once surgical privileges are granted, hospitals have several ways to monitor the surgical staff.

- Surgical complications and deaths are discussed at weekly or biweekly Morbidity and Mortality (M&M) conferences. No other single feature of local peer review is as effective in maintaining good surgical practice as standing up in front of an audience of your colleagues and attempting to explain a poor surgical result. Everyone learns, not only from one's own personal errors but also from the shared mistakes of others. Recurring complications and persistently poor results exposed in M&M conferences often result in more formal review of a surgeon's practice.
- Members of the Tissue Committee review all of the material sent to the pathology department from the operating room. Cases in which normal tissue or no tissue at all is removed are subjected to particularly close scrutiny. Each case is judged with regard to the necessity for surgery, as well as its outcome.
- Surgeons whose work is criticized too frequently at M&M conferences or by the Tissue Committee may be referred for investigation to the hospital's Surgical Quality Assurance Committee. At these hearings, accused surgeons can be represented by

counsel and have the right to examine and try to refute the case against them. If the practice review demonstrates inferior care, the Surgical Quality Assurance Committee may recommend censure, limitation of practice, or even revocation of hospital and operating privileges. The committee makes its recommendations to the hospital administration, where the final decision rests. If an adverse action is taken, hospitals are required by law to notify the Medical Licensing Board.

State Supervision

Perhaps the most important agencies for controlling the quality of medicine and surgery in this country are the State Medical Licensing Boards. Every state has such a board, which, unlike the professional associations, has as its primary concern the protection and the welfare of the public.

Since a license to practice medicine is required of every doctor in all 50 states, suspension or revocation of a state medical license is an effective measure for controlling impaired, incompetent, or unethical physicians. State medical licensing boards have the power to award, deny, limit, suspend, or revoke a license to practice medicine. Grounds for those adverse actions include malpractice, incompetence, addiction to alcohol or drugs, negligence, conviction of a felony, narcotics violations, fraud (including Medicare, Medicaid, insurance, and mail fraud), mental illness, unprofessional conduct, and disciplinary actions taken against the medical practitioner by other states.

While most of the cases investigated by state boards come to them as a result of reports from local hospitals and the public, many state boards have broad investigative powers and need not wait for someone to report undesirable physicians. Active monitoring of drug use and prescription excess, as well as close communication with drug and alcohol dependence facilities, are common mechanisms to identify impaired physicians before the quality of their medical or surgical care deteriorates. The state licensing board also has the power to force the impaired physician to cease to practice, and can assist the physician in entering an approved rehabilitation center, where progress is closely monitored.

Not all states have such active medical licensing boards. Funding of broad investigative and regulatory powers is difficult to obtain in many states. More widespread appreciation by the public of the important functions performed by these state licensing boards could create enough political pressure to ensure adequate funding.

The individual licensing boards operate independently, but they share information at the national level through the Federation of State Medical Boards. The Federation has established a national Disciplinary Data Bank (DDB). The DDB is a central computerized repository for collecting, recording, and distributing to all appropriate agencies data on formal disciplinary actions taken against physicians by any board, hospital, or other authority. Since the establishment of the DDB, it is no longer possible for a physician to be censored in one location and move to another location and resume practice.

Another powerful tool of the state medical licensing boards is reregistration. Licenses to practice are granted for a specified period, usually one to three years. At the end of that time, the physician must apply for a renewal. The applicant is queried about any censoring actions, arrests, malpractice suits, or any other sanctions taken against him or her since the previous application. This information is added to the DDB. Failure to provide factual information is grounds for revocation of the medical license. Without a license, it is a felony to practice medicine or surgery.

While state boards are becoming more successful in finding impaired physicians, incompetence is less easily identified. Malpractice cases must be reported to the DDB and are investigated for evidence of incompetence, censoring actions taken by local hospitals are reviewed, charges of incompetence brought by medical colleagues and the public are given close attention, but despite such measures, incompetence characterizes only a small fraction of the total number of disciplinary cases.

How well does this surveillance system work? As of mid-1990, there were more than 27,000 entries against over 15,000 physicians lodged in the DDB. This amounts to 3 percent of the nation's 550,000 physicians, a figure considerably less than the 10 to 15 percent of physicians estimated to be impaired or incompetent.

The DDB has been in operation only since 1982. In 1986, there were 2,302 formal disciplinary actions, a 37 percent increase over the total for 1984. In 1993, the Federation of State Medical Boards reported that states had revoked the licenses of 1,176 physicians, restricted the practices of 1,001, penalized or reprimanded 811, and taken nonprejudicial action against 630, for a total of 3,618 disciplinary actions. Although this represents a 10 percent increase in the overall number of actions compared with 1992, it still represents adverse actions against only 6 doctors out of every 1,000. The Federation of State Medical Licensing Boards estimates that for every disciplinary action that results in formal charges, there are at least 10 to 15 "informal" hearings that are not included in the DDB. These hearings, concerned with less serious charges, are also powerful modifiers of physician behavior. It seems fair to conclude that the mechanisms for surveillance and enforcement are in place at the state level, but more actions could be taken. Adequate funding may permit expansion of these programs.

All of the 50 state medical societies have established programs to rehabilitate impaired physicians. Each also offers programs in CME to provide opportunities for physicians to keep up with the latest developments in medical practice. Those programs, however, are primarily oriented toward assisting the physician, not the public. Furthermore, they are voluntary.

Federal Oversight

A number of federal agencies police the medical profession. Through the Health Care Financing Administration (HCFA), a division of the Department of Health and Human Services, the federal government administers the Professional Review Organizations (PROs), review boards composed of physicians and laypersons.

Federal PROs are established in each federal district to monitor the quality of care given to the 37 million patients who receive Medicare. The PROs can recommend to the Office of the Inspector General (OIG) that physicians guilty of "gross and flagrant" negligence be barred from participation in the Medicare program, or that fines be levied against them. Since 1986, only 262 physicians have been recommended for sanction by the regional PROs. By the end of 1993, the OIG had acted on those recommendations by barring 118 physicians from participation in Medicare and fining 28. The federal PRO program is still evolving, but judging from the small number of physicians sanctioned, it seems to be more valuable as a deterrent to overcharging and fraud than a means for weeding out incompetent or impaired physicians.

The Health Quality Improvement Act (PL 99-660), passed by Congress in 1986, established a national clearinghouse for information relating to malpractice, disciplinary actions, adverse findings by professional societies, and changes in hospital privileges for individual physicians. All medical liability insurance carriers, state medical boards, and health-care institutions must report such actions to the agency. Hospitals must request information from the clearinghouse whenever a physician applies for privileges. Unfortunately, several start-up problems have limited the effectiveness of this federal data bank. In essence, however, the federal clearinghouse duplicates many of the functions well handled in the voluntary sphere by the Federation of State Medical Boards' Disciplinary Data Bank.

Two national organizations have assumed the watchdog role for surgery. The American College of Surgeons, through its Central Judiciary Committee, can censure, suspend, or revoke fellowship in the college. Such actions are taken whenever a fellow is disciplined for any reason by a hospital, state licensing board, or court. Loss of fellowship privileges also occurs whenever the Judiciary Committee finds evidence of moral turpitude or unethical practices, such as fee splitting, kickbacks, "ghost" surgery (billing for surgery someone else actually does), itinerant surgery (delegating postoperative care), or charging unreasonable fees. In the past several years, the number of surgeons disciplined by the College has tripled, although College membership grew only slightly. The increase in the number of disciplinary actions has been attributed to more effective means of gathering information.

Some of the national specialty boards deny recertification to physicians whose professional conduct has resulted in some formal disciplinary action. Since many certificates of specialization are time-limited and require periodic examinations to maintain currency, refusal to renew is an effective deterrent. No specialty board has yet advocated actually revoking certification for a disciplined physician, despite the fact that the courts have consistently upheld the right of a private organization to enforce reasonable rules regarding continued membership.

It is important to note that the specialty boards and the College of Surgeons police only the most qualified surgeons, those who are board certified and those who are fellows of the ACS. Less qualified surgeons do not have such supervision—even more reason for patients to choose a surgeon with the best qualifications.

The American Medical Association has long been concerned with physician impairment and incompetence. Rather than adopting a regulatory role, however, the AMA has concentrated on alerting the public and the profession to the dangers of impairment and incompetence. The AMA has funded numerous studies of physician impairment, published reports, and sponsored seminars on these problems. It has assisted state and federal legislatures in formulating laws and regulations, and it has strongly condemned unethical behavior .

The overwhelming majority of physicians in this country are intellectually competent, have a strong ethical system, and practice skillful medicine. Physicians are increasingly accepting the responsibility for self-policing and initiating actions against colleagues who are incompetent or impaired. Since few other professions can match the extent and breadth of existing regulatory agencies for quality assurance, individual identification remains the key.

EPILOGUE

America's health-care system is in turmoil. Never before have problems of such magnitude confronted both medical professionals and the public.

The principal problem facing American medicine today is the seemingly inexorable escalation in the overall cost of health care. Multiple attempts at cost control have previously been made at the federal, state, and local levels, without appreciable effect. To most careful observers, it has become increasingly clear that only a complete overhaul of our current health care system will control costs.

How the intertwined problems of cost, universal access to health care for all citizens, and malpractice litigation are resolved will affect present and future generations of Americans. At this point in time, no one can predict what type of system will ultimately be adopted, or precisely how the new system will affect everyone. It is *extremely* important for you to become knowledgeable about the merits and limitations of the various health care plans that have been, and will be, proposed.

To enable you to compare competing proposals for health care reform, it is helpful to view health care as a triangle composed of equal and mutually dependent sides: quality, access, and cost. In this analogy, it is not possible to maximize all three sides simultaneously; highest quality, universal access, and lowest cost cannot be made to coexist. Although it is theoretically possible to design a compromise equilibrium among these three components, hard decisions will need to be made seeking those compromises that would be acceptable to the American public.

That's why it's important to become informed about specific proposals for changing our health care system. People should ask themselves which sides of the triangle are being compromised and find out how those compromises will affect them. Remember, despite any claims to the contrary, no system will be perfect.

Whatever system of health care is eventually chosen, it will become *our* system, whether or not everyone is in agreement. Clearly, now is the time for Americans to become involved and communicate with their legislators.

INDEX